The Patient's Guide to the Complete Medical Examination and the Prevention of Medical Errors

SHELDON COHEN M.D. F.A.C.P.

iUniverse, Inc.
New York Lincoln Shanghai

The Patient's Guide to the Complete Medical Examination and the Prevention of Medical Errors

iUniverse books may be ordered through booksellers or by contacting:

iUniverse
2021 Pine Lake Road, Suite 100
Lincoln, NE 68512
www.iuniverse.com
1-800-Authors (1-800-288-4677)

The information, ideas, and suggestions in this book are not intended as a substitute for professional medical advice. Before following any suggestions contained in this book, you should consult your personal physician. Neither the author nor the publisher shall be liable or responsible for any loss or damage allegedly arising as a consequence of your use or application of any information or suggestions in this book.

ISBN-13: 978-0-595-42662-1 (pbk)
ISBN-13: 978-0-595-68174-7 (cloth)
ISBN-13: 978-0-595-86990-9 (ebk)
ISBN-10: 0-595-42662-X (pbk)
ISBN-10: 0-595-68174-3 (cloth)
ISBN-10: 0-595-86990-4 (ebk)

Printed in the United States of America

The Patient's Guide
to the Complete
Medical Examination and the
Prevention
of Medical Errors

To physician's best teachers—the patient

CONTENTS

Part III   Laboratory Data

Part IV   Summary

Part V   The Prevention Of Medical Errors

Part VI   Medical Resources

INTRODUCTION

When you get a complete medical examination you are taking an important first step in safeguarding your health. Learn what you are about to go through. Ask questions, read, surf the net. You must be an active participant in this important process. You are a critical part of the team whose goal is to see that you will be correctly diagnosed and treated.

This book is a guide to a complete medical examination (a medical history, physical examination and basic laboratory data). This is not a book for medical professionals. It is a book for you, the patient. I will attempt to answer the questions that have been asked of me over the years as the medical history is taken and the physical examination is performed. You need to know why the physician asks the questions he does, what can be learned from a thorough physical examination, how the data is put together to arrive at the proper diagnosis, and how this information will enable you to contribute to the prevention of medical errors.

The latest emphasis on minimizing medical errors is involving the patient. Being an educated patient is your best defense. It starts with knowing your state of health. I can't emphasize this enough, and when you do learn all you can about your mental and physical body, you can be of major assistance to your doctors and nurses and other healthcare team members in providing optimal and safe care for you. Granted, this may all take time and presumes you are an ambulatory patient with the time to spend evaluating your options, but the time needed may not be available if you are involved in an acute life and death medical or surgical situation and you are in an unfamiliar medical environment. If that is the case, a written summary of your medical history—kept on your person or otherwise easily available—can be very helpful. In the absence of this information, and if you or a significant other are unable to provide good clinical information, you must trust the professionals that find themselves in the very difficult and responsible position of having your life suddenly thrust in their hands.

There are many ways you can provide valuable input to your healthcare provider and protect yourself from an untoward event—and they will be discussed later, but first we will discuss the important first step for you to take in safeguarding your health: that is to learn all you can by getting a complete medical examination—the main subject of this book.

This book is a guide to what you should expect when you present yourself to your physician, or other qualified health care professional, for the purpose of undergoing the complete medical examination. By qualified healthcare professional, I mean a primary care physician (internal medicine, pediatrics and family practice), a nurse or physician assistant. For the purpose of this book I will use the word "physician" when I write about the professional taking your medical history and performing your physical examination. More often than not the word physician will mean a doctor of medicine (M.D.). Also, an ever increasing number of physicians are women, but I will use the masculine "he" as opposed to he or she or (s)he. This is strictly for ease of typing. The "he" means a male or female physician, or in some cases a nurse or physician's assistant.

Physicians—doctors of medicine—first learn how to evaluate a patient in their early years of medical school. By the time budding physicians have graduated, they have had experience in taking medical histories and completely examining patients under close senior M.D. supervision. At this juncture, medical students have learned how to learn, and only a continuing experience will allow them to polish their craft. Nurses can receive Master's Degree specialized training in the performance of the complete medical examination, and physician assistants can be trained as well.

In the 1920's the Metropolitan Life Insurance Company demonstrated that policyholders who underwent annual complete medical examinations lived longer than those who did not. On the strength of these statistics the American Medical Association recommended periodic examinations of all healthy persons starting at age thirty-five. The implementation of this recommendation has not been uniformly applied. Corporate executives have utilized the concept extensively, while the average person has failed to receive a *complete* medical examination in any great numbers.

There are those who argue against the periodic complete medical examination, saying that it may not be cost effective in terms of the yield. They propose that the evaluation of patients who have no symptoms should be selective and based upon the age and sex of the patient. This approach has been endorsed by major medical organizations in the United States and Canada. Physicians do not dispute the wisdom of these endorsements, but cling to the belief that the complete medical examination is important—and they cite the following reasons:

1.   Patients expect a complete medical examination.

2. Physicians have had numerous experiences where the performance of the complete medical examination has elicited unexpected critical findings.

3. A carefully done complete medical examination has an important role in the physician-patient relationship. Anything that fosters a close relationship between the physician and patient will promote understanding and minimize the possibility of medical errors.

4. The complete medical examination offers patients the best opportunity to learn whether you have health risks that must be followed. A full understanding of these risks will allow you to take charge of your own health.

5. In these days of high malpractice litigation, the complete medical examination offers protection for both the physician and the patient. One of the most important reasons for malpractice suits is failure to diagnose. The structured complete medical examination can reduce lawsuits filed for this reason.

I am a strong advocate of both of these approaches: selective evaluation and the complete medical examination.

Is there anything wrong with the complete medical examination? The major difficulty is its cost. It takes the physicians' time and costs the patients' money. This is where the well trained nurse and physician's assistant can help. Another problem is the number of false-positive tests that must be evaluated. When these tests are invasive there is slight risk to you the patient.

The most a physician can say to you after successful completion of the full examination is that, "Your examination is completely normal." There is a certain amount of reassurance in that statement, but inherent within it is that there is no guarantee. You will be told that it is impossible to predict exactly what the future holds, but if you follow preventive recommendations, you will reduce your risks for death or disability. Patients understand this and are appreciative of the reassurance they can get upon conclusion of the complete medical examination.

Finally, with this book, I will attempt to answer my patient's questions asked of me throughout my medical career. We will go through a medical history and a complete physical examination just as I have done with medical students in my private office and in the hospital. I will give clinical examples after each section. These examples, illustrating the history or physical examination point discussed, have been taken from my own and colleagues experiences. There will also be

some examples of unusual cases of great clinical and human interest. I hope that
when we have finished, you will have a better understanding of the art and sci-
ence of history taking, the technique of performing a thorough physical examination, the importance of basic laboratory studies, the necessity of putting all the
information together in an accurate and clearly understandable manner, and the
importance of storing the information in a place where instant call-up is available. Once you are firm and secure in understanding your medical condition, you
are in an excellent position to use the information in a positive way to take charge
of your health.

PART I
THE MEDICAL HISTORY

✦

"Let the patient talk, doctor, she's trying to tell you the diagnosis."

Sir William Osler
(1849–1919)

INTRODUCTION

It has been estimated that a well-taken medical history will provide the diagnosis eighty percent of the time. From actual experience I would confirm this statement. Sir William Osler, the greatest diagnostician and medical educator of his time, thought enough of this statistic to verbalize the quotation on the preceding page. These simple words should be the first assertion made to new medical students. They will diagnose more from a well-taken medical history then they will diagnose from all the technological wizardry developed in the twenty and twenty-first century. The capturing of medical history information is vital to learn about your health status. What are your symptoms? What is the chronology of events? What can the physician learn from your history in order to zero in effectively on your diagnosis and treatment? The medical history is your chance to develop rapport and a working relationship with your physician and health care team. You need to be assured that everything is done to carefully elicit all the pertinent medical information so vital to your physician's ability to correctly diagnose and treat. Once your physician collects this important historical information, he will combine it with objective data acquired from a well-performed physical examination and laboratory data.

HISTORY ACQUISITION METHODS

There is more than one way to get a medical history:

(1) Experienced physician (M.D.)

The most optimal is an experienced physician well versed in the natural history of disease who skillfully probes with well-worded questions geared to your symptoms. You should be allowed to tell your story with a minimum of interruptions. Learning the art of history taking requires more skill and knowledge than learning the art of the mostly mechanical acts of the physical examination. It takes a while for young physicians, raised in this high tech milieu, to appreciate this truism.

(2) Computer

The next method for acquiring a complete medical history is by use of a computer. The first such efforts were developed by Dr. Warner Slack who prior to 1970 did his pioneering work at the University of Wisconsin. He is currently at Beth Israel Deaconess Hospital in Boston, Massachusetts. In 1970 I attended a post graduate course given by Dr. Slack and was so enamored by this development that I and a friend of mine (a computer expert) developed a computerized medical history system. In those days laptop or desktop computers did not exist. But we did manage to work with a new development that consisted of a primitive desktop that had a cassette tape with the history questions that fit into a slot on the 'machine'. The questions appeared on a 'cathode ray' tube screen, and the patients answered by pressing either a yes, a no, a don't know, or a don't understand key. If the answer was no, the patient went on to the next question. If the answer was yes, the follow up questions branched into more detail. The answers were put on another tape, which was sent over a telephone line to a central computer filling a large climate controlled room. The answers were collated by the computer and returned again via teletype to my office. You ended up with a completely typed medical history varying in size from two to five pages depending upon the number of yes responses. You had the additional assurance that all the questions previously programmed into the history had to be asked and answered. This guaranteed a uniform questioning format for all the patients who utilized the system. I put 1500 patients on the 'machine' (see appendix). A questionnaire filled out by all participating patients revealed that ninety-five percent viewed it favorably. Physicians, however, viewed it unfavorably—feeling as if a machine was replacing them. I remember at the time being told that "if you keep this up you'll put yourself out of work." I was also told by the technical people involved that, "it won't be long and we'll be able to do this out of a little box sitting on your desk." Although this system was not accepted by the medical profession at the time, this type of development has led to an electronic medical record that hopefully will some day replace the paper record. Progress is being made slowly and carefully by pioneers such as Dr. Warner Slack.

(3) Nurse or physician assistant

With proper training and experience, these highly trained professionals can do an excellent job of history acquisition.

(4) Paper Questionnaire

The fourth method is the paper history form where questions are printed, and the patients are requested to fill out the form. This is in widespread use and is viewed as a fair method of history acquisition. The patient spends the time recording the data. A well-designed form can elicit valuable information. Most of the forms do not have the capability to branch logically once a yes response is given, so those detailed queries must remain the province of the physician taking your history, using the printed form as a guide.

These latter three methods are recognition of the importance of a good history, and also recognition of the fact that the busy physician, strapped for time, could use help in its acquisition.

Now we'll get into the details of the medical history.

BIOGRAPHICAL DATA

This is the first information obtained in the medical history. You will document this usually on a paper form, or you may be asked directly. The necessary information includes your name, sex, age, date of birth, address, phone number, birthplace, marital status, race and ethnic origin. Some of this information could have important bearing on your health history.

CLINICAL EXAMPLES

A fifteen-year-old boy developed abdominal pain associated with a temperature of 102. The pain started in the right lower part of his abdomen and then spread diffusely throughout his entire belly. He was placed in the hospital with the presumptive diagnosis of appendicitis, but his symptoms resolved before he was to be operated upon and he was sent home. Four months later he had another attack, which again quickly resolved. A final and unusual diagnosis was subsequently made, based upon the region of the world his mother and father came from, and the fact that a member of his family had been diagnosed with the illness. His family was from North Africa, and this illness, a genetic one, is seen in North African Arabs, Sephardic Jews, Turks, Greeks and Italians. It is known as familial Mediterranean fever. This condition is caused by a defect on a specific gene. He was started on therapy and did well.

This is an example of how the biographical data (origin and ethnicity) led to the proper diagnosis.

A young African-American man developed severe pain in his lower legs, his lumbar spine and his abdomen. He was in great distress. The diagnosis of sickle cell anemia was suspected. This condition is seen almost exclusively in African Americans, and the characteristic findings on his complete blood count led to the diagnosis. Sickle cell anemia is a hereditary condition where red blood cells, instead of being the normal round shape, are shaped like a sickle. These abnormal cells can clog blood capillaries causing a variety of symptoms. Proper therapy has greatly prolonged life in these patients.

It was the patient's race, in this instance, that led to a proper diagnosis.

CHIEF COMPLAINT

Patient's own words or medical clarification

The chief complaint is the initiation of the medical history. It is the reason you have visited the doctor. You should be encouraged to volunteer information in your own words. If you become too wordy and wander off into tangents, your physician should keep firm control over the direction of the interview.

"I'm here for a complete examination."

"I developed some chest pain"

"My back hurts."

"I'm having constant diarrhea"

"I'm getting short of breath."

You may have one or more of such symptoms to relate. If the physician can rely on your exact words then the chief complaint is written in the chart verbatim. If your words are ambiguous, or the physician is in anyway unsure of your meaning, then after careful clarification the words should be put into medical language. It is important that you are allowed to describe your problem with as little interruption as possible. You should be allowed to speak freely, and the physician should avoid leading questions. Remember Dr. Osler—you're trying to tell your doctor the diagnosis.

Tabulate complaints separately

The physician has to be certain that all chief complaints are collected and tabulated each on a separate line. They also have to be sure that all the information is collected by asking finally, "Are there any other symptoms that brought you here today?" "Do you have any other concerns?" "Any other complaints?" It may be that some of the chief complaint may be uncovered in the subsequent interview after the initial chief complaint has been obtained.

Duration

The duration of each symptom should be listed adjacent to the symptom: Chest pain—one month. Low back pain—five days. Diarrhea—three weeks. Shortness of breath—two weeks.

CLINICAL EXAMPLES

Sometimes the first sentence of a patient's medical history is enough for a physician to make a diagnosis. "I fell weak. I lost ten pounds and I'm thirsty all the time." The diagnosis of Diabetes Mellitus was confirmed by a quick urinalysis test followed by a blood sugar test.

In this instance the three facts of the chief complaint led to a presumptive diagnosis, quickly proven by the follow-up tests.

"It feels like an elephant stepped on my chest." The patient had what sounded like angina—chest pain due to a blocked coronary artery or arteries. Coronary artery angiography was confirmatory. His anterior descending coronary artery was almost completely blocked. He underwent successful cardiac surgery.

The diagnosis was made by the patient's classical description of angina pectoris (cardiac pain) given in the chief complaint. Other diagnosis may be responsible for such a description by the patient, but the first and most important cause must be considered to be cardiac and ruled out immediately.

Many years ago as an intern at Cook County Hospital's Fantus Clinic, on a follow up visit, a patient's chief complaint was, "I'm not any better. I couldn't take the stuff you prescribed."

"Why?"

"Well, I managed to swallow those big pills, but trying to get that liquid down was impossible—yuck."

No wonder. This was not exactly the route I had in mind when I prescribed vaginal suppositories and a vinegar douche.

This therapeutic foul-up highlights a recent study done that determined as many as a third of patients forget or misunderstand or fail to read the prescription instructions. It is always best to know the name of the medicine (both generic and trade name), the exact dose and frequency and duration before leaving the doctors office. Don't trust your memory—write it down.

PRESENT ILLNESS

Introduction

The present illness is the heart of the medical history. It amplifies the chief complaint and clarifies its relationship to other symptoms you may be experiencing, or any events of significance that may bear a relationship to your chief complaint. Such clarification is important in leading to a presumptive diagnosis. The physician should start the present illness by asking, "Tell me about what brings you to see me," or "Give me your story, please." This portion of the medical history is where the symptoms are clarified in detail. The present illness should tell a story:

Does it convey a clear picture about the extent of your distress?

How has the illness affected you physically?

How has it impacted your family?

Has the problem or problems interfered with your work?

Has it impacted your finances?

What has been the psychological impact?

The written description should be legible and as brief as possible for the benefit of the physician and all caregivers involved with your future care. This is easy when the symptoms are clear-cut and lead to a single diagnosis, but can be much more complicated when in spite of continuous questioning the diagnosis is obscure. If the latter is the case, then further questioning of a negative and positive nature must continue. Only then can the physician get as close as possible to a firm presumptive diagnosis based upon your history alone.

Duration

Although the duration of your symptoms have been included in the chief complaint, it may be appropriate to amplify the details in the present illness, particularly in light of the symptom's degrees of severity over time.

Nature of the symptoms:

Location, severity, character, radiation, timing, aggravating factors, precipitating factors, relieving factors, setting, quantity, medication taken, helpful or not, associated symptoms, patient's perception.

Each symptom must be clarified and quantified as to severity and character. It is with experience and knowledge of disease that the physician can learn the important questions to ask. Take chest pain for example. It is not enough to know that you are experiencing chest pain. The location must be defined as precisely as possible. Has trauma been involved? The physician should ask you to put your finger on where it hurts, as a means of precisely locating the site. You should be asked to quantify the pain. On a scale of one to ten—with ten being the worst and one the least—put a number on your pain. Does your pain stay where specified, or does it move (radiate) to other locations such as the back, the shoulders, one or both arms, the upper abdomen, or the jaw and teeth? What is the duration of the pain? Does it last for seconds, or minutes, or hours, or is it constant? How would you describe the pain? The physician should give examples. Sharp, dull like a toothache, piercing, burning, pressure. Does the pain interfere with your daily activities? What aggravates the pain? Position? Movement? Physical exercise? Breathing? Heavy lifting? Is the pain increased with exertion? Does it go away with rest? Is the pain associated with other symptoms such as cold sweat, nausea, vomiting, shortness of breath?

It is with queries such as above that the physician will be well on the way to arriving at an accurate diagnosis. Regardless of the nature of the symptom, detailed questioning by an experienced and knowledgeable physician can narrow the diagnostic options. This can be cost-effective as well, because a thorough history (and physical examination) allows the physician to pinpoint the necessary tests needed for confirmatory purposes.

CLINICAL EXAMPLES

The patient's chief complaint was "bad headache." Details of the present illness revealed that these headaches awakened the patient in the middle of the night. The pain was severe, one-sided and described as being "around the right eye and in front of and above the ear." It lasted about an hour. Also associated with the pain was a flood of tears from the effected eye. These details were enough to make the diagnosis of cluster headaches. It is an illness of unknown etiology, but is amenable to acute and long term preventive therapy.

Here again is another example of the chief complaint yielding a prompt and correct diagnosis.

The patient's chief complaint was "having trouble hearing." The details of the present illness revealed that she first realized that she was experiencing this difficulty when she found that she had to turn her head to understand what people were saying. The onset of this symptom seemed to be rather abrupt. She also noted persistent ringing in the involved ear (tinnitus), a feeling of fullness, some loss of equilibrium and headache. All these details were suspicious for the diagnosis of acoustic neuroma, a tumor of the eighth cranial, or acoustic nerve. Her tumor was small and was successfully removed with surgery.

On the other hand, here's what could happen when you don't take a careful present illness. As a young intern I was working a twelve hour shift in Chicago's Cook County Hospital's emergency department. This was a solid twelve hours of work, as I never remember the waiting room emptying out. A middle-aged man's chief complaint was that he was "having trouble with my nose." We spent much of our time in this busy location taking direct care of patients and also triaging many patients to the proper medical clinic where they can get more acute specialized care. In this case, during an exceptionally busy time, I told the patient that we would send him to the Ear Nose and Throat clinic where he would be taken care of. About an hour later the ENT resident came down to the emergency room and told me to come to the ENT clinic so I could see the man I sent to him with the "nose trouble." When we arrived, the patient was seated on the examining table, stooped over with his hands on his lap. The resident spoke to the patient and said, "Tell this doctor about your nose, sir." The patient picked up his head slowly and responded, "Well you see, doc, my nose keeps getting longer and longer until it gets all the way out here." The patient extended his right arm full length forward. "And then it gets so heavy I fall over." That story just didn't stop there. My good friend—the ENT resident—spread it around the hospital. All I could hope is that others, as well as myself, learned the importance of a carefully taken present illness. Yes, the patient belatedly got the right referral—to the psychiatric department.

PAST HISTORY

Introduction

Here is where the physician attempts to discover if there has been any change in your normal living pattern as a result of the recent problem or problems. "Now I'm going to ask you questions about your past health." There are specific areas that must be evaluated. You should be asked the perception of your general health. Has there been any change in overall strength or mental status? Has there been any change in the pattern of living? Have there been any unusual activities before the onset of your current problem? Has your weight remained stable, or has there been any weight gain or loss? Do you get a good night's sleep, or is there a disturbance in the sleep pattern?

The aspects of the past history to investigate are the following:

Allergies

Do you have Asthma, hay fever, food allergies, or hives? Are you allergic to any medicines? If the response is positive this will require clarification necessitating further questioning: Have you ever experienced a reaction such as skin rash, hives, itching, fainting, wheezing, or shortness of breath?

Has there ever been an anaphylactic reaction to any medication or dye. This is a serious life-threatening reaction where one goes into shock immediately after receiving the offending agent (a medication or an imaging study dye or an insect sting). If this is the case, appropriate warnings must be placed on your records as repeat use of the offending agent could result in serious consequences.

Has the use of any medication caused a reaction such as anemia, bleeding, bruising, gastrointestinal disturbances including nausea, vomiting, diarrhea, or abdominal pain? Have any medications caused palpitations, headache, or dizziness?

You should be asked specifically if you are allergic to penicillin, sulfa, any other antibiotic, aspirin, or any other medication. If a medication allergy has been identified, the information must be placed on a prominent place on the

13

chart (the front cover), or computer record where it is easily available for all personnel to see. Serious problems could result by the failure to remember such vital information. Anyone who has a significant medication or dye allergy should be encouraged to wear an identification bracelet naming the offending agent. It should be noted that the use of prescription and over-the-counter drugs sends more people to the emergency room than cocaine. These statistics were released in 2006 by the Substance Abuse and Mental health Services Administration (SAMHSA) and reflect 2004 data. One in four—or 495,732—drug related emergency room visits involved pharmaceuticals: prescription or over-the-counter drugs. One in five visits—383,350—involved cocaine. Marijuana caused 215,665 visits. The medications you take, including over-the-counter medications and herbs, must be known. They could be the cause of your problem.

Acute infectious diseases

Questions should be asked about whether you ever had the usual childhood diseases such as measles, mumps, German measles, chicken pox, whooping cough, or scarlet fever. Has there been a history of pneumonia, tuberculosis, pleurisy, acute rheumatic fever, rheumatic heart disease, hepatitis, poliomyelitis, tropical or parasitic diseases? Have you ever experienced any sexually transmitted disease such as chlamydia, gonorrhea, syphilis, venereal warts, or HIV? Any other infectious disease not discussed? The chronic nature of some of these illnesses may have bearing in later life and could be impacting your present illness.

Immunizations

Past immunizations, if known, must be recorded—with dates if available. The dates are important to determine if there is any need for a booster shot. The immunizations include measles, mumps, chickenpox, whooping cough (pertussis), tetanus, rubella, hepatitis B, hepatitis A, polio, pneumococcal pneumonia, influenza, PPD (TB skin test), and its result (positive or negative). Were there any unusual reactions to any of these immunizations?

Past Medical History

The physician should ask if you have ever received medical care. If so, what were the problems or issues that were addressed? Sometimes you may not remember specific details of past care, so the physician can refresh your memory by asking specifically whether you have had any X-rays, CAT scans, MRI's, blood tests, electrocardiograms, or other special tests. To jog your memory about past medical problems it may be necessary to ask, "Have you ever been under a doctor's care for any specific medical problem? Have you taken or do you take any medications for a specific medical problem?" By carefully evaluating the past medical history it may be possible to uncover clues that will aid in diagnosing the current problem(s).

Past Surgical History

Have you ever had any surgical operation under local anesthesia or spinal anesthesia or general anesthesia? If so, what was the procedure and the date? What is the name of the hospital or office in which it was performed? Who was the surgeon? What was the outcome? Were there any complications either during or after the surgery? Were there any anesthetic complications? Have you ever received any blood transfusions?

Past Traumatic History

Have you ever been in any major accidents requiring medical or surgical or orthopedic care? It is important to know if there was ever a history of unconsciousness from a head injury, for complications such as a hematoma (collection of blood on the brain) can present with unusual symptoms. Have you ever experienced any fractures? Are there any resulting disabilities from any of these injuries?

Medications

It is vital to know what medications you are taking. The precise name and current dose and the frequency of all medications must be recorded. It is also important to be sure that you are taking the medication precisely as ordered, as sometimes failure to respond to therapy could be traced to taking the medication incorrectly. This information may be crucial to the determination of the treatment's efficacy and possible need for adjustments. Should doses of the medication be missed, the physician needs to understand why. Are the reasons cognitive? Is it financial? Are you too busy and you forget? Are you experiencing side effects? Whatever the cause, help should be offered in remedying it—as it may be important to your overall health.

As previously mentioned, patients are frequently using herbs and/or over the counter medications. It is important to know if you are taking any of these, as it is possible that there could be medication-herb interactions.

Drug-food interactions can also occur and this has to be considered by the physician, especially if you are having unusual side effects.

Other Drug Use

The physician should question you about the use of any illegal drugs. One cannot determine who is at risk by appearance alone. You should be made to understand that the questions are not for the purpose of making any judgment, but is rather for identifying risk factors for diseases such as hepatitis and HIV. If you are uncomfortable answering such questions, the wise physician will not push the issue. You may be more forthcoming at a later date after you have gotten more comfortable in the physician's presence.

Statistics gathered in 2003 demonstrated that for persons twelve years of age and older, 8.2% used an illegal drug. 6.2% used marijuana. 2.7% used a psycho-therapeutic drug for a non-medical use. By numbers this means that 14.7 million people have used marijuana, 6.3 million have used a prescription drug for a non-medical use, 2.3 million have used cocaine, 1 million have used hallucinogens, 570,000 have used inhalants and 119,000 have used heroin.

With statistics such as these, the physician should eventually determine if there has been any illegal drug use, especially if there is a strong possibility it can have impact upon, or be the cause of the symptoms described in the Chief Complaint or the Present Illness.

Obstetric History

The number of pregnancies, miscarriages and abortions should be determined. Have there been any difficult pregnancies or labor? Have you ever undergone a Cesarean Section? What were the dates and place of delivery? Was there a history of toxemia of pregnancy or any other pregnancy or post pregnancy complication? Where there any complications involving the newborn?

Sexual History

Although an uncomfortable area to question, this could be important and should be pursued. What is the degree of sexual activity if any? Are you involved in a stable relationship? What is your sexual preference? What means of birth control, if any, are used?

CLINICAL EXAMPLES

In the early days of the discovery of HIV, when only homosexuals were being diagnosed with the disease, a man came into my office complaining of a sore mouth. It was clear he had thrush (an infection of the mouth caused by a yeast organism known as candida albicans). I asked him about his sexual preference. He told me he was homosexual. An HIV test was ordered and was positive. Since these early days HIV has become an international health problem affecting anyone regardless of sexual preference.

A twenty-one year old male was brought to the emergency room by ambulance. He was in status epilepticus (unremitting seizure). After specific therapy his seizure was finally resolved. He had no idea how he had gotten to the hospital, nor what had happened to him. He denied ever having had a seizure before. The initial impression in a man with sudden onset of a first seizure would be a brain tumor, but further questioning failed to reveal any other symptoms suggestive of this diagnosis. Nevertheless, that did not rule it out, and it was recommended that he undergo tests to determine if this was the diagnosis. He had no recollection of his pre-seizure activities. A day went by and his memory returned, and on being questioned again about immediate pre-seizure recollections, his eyes opened wide. "Oh God, I remember," he said. "I shot up cocaine for the first time." That made the diagnosis. I asked him if he was a religious man. "Not really," he said. I suggested, however, that he should go to the church of his choice and thank God that he was alive. Any repetition of the same behavior, based upon what happened his first time, could mean he might be performing the last act of his life. He was very grateful—and one could only pray he learned his lesson.

FAMILY HISTORY

Definition

A family medical history is a record of the illnesses that are prevalent in the family and thus may directly impact your well being. This is one of the most critical areas of the entire history. By careful and detailed questioning, the physician may be able to determine what health risks might be in your future. Once this information is obtained, proper advice can be provided to minimize the risk.

Heritable illnesses

In terms of heritable illnesses, it is important that you are asked specific details about the illnesses that have affected your mother and father, sisters, brothers, aunts, uncles, and cousins. The cause of your relative's death and the age of death may bear importantly on your own future illness or mortality. Those illnesses that have the most impact are diabetes mellitus, colon polyps, hypertension, coronary artery disease, congenital disorders and, certain cancers. In addition to learning about these illnesses it is crucial to determine the age when the relative was afflicted. If age forty, the significance is distinctly greater than if age seventy-five, because the age of forty would strongly suggest a genetic predisposition, whereas age seventy-five may not.

How used

A specific diagnosis may possibly be made from family history data.

The history can help to determine the exact type of medical testing that may be diagnostic for the disease in question.

Statistics may determine your risk of certain diseases.

Statistics may determine the chance of passing the problem to your children.

You can be educated to avoid or prepare for the illness in question.

What it can't do

It can't precisely predict your future, but it is currently the best guess we have. At the least, knowing your future risk may encourage you to change your behavior.

If your family is small, the family history is less likely to provide statistically significant information upon which to predict your future.

It doesn't apply, of course, if you are adopted and not aware of your biological parents.

The future

With the completion of the genome mapping project and the future ability to map one's DNA, it may be possible to predict all of the diseases you may fall prey to. Until that time, however, the family history gives your physician the best possible look into your future.

CLINICAL EXAMPLES

A pale, short teenager complained of fatigue and easy bruising. Anemia was confirmed by a blood count. He also had a low platelet count, which explained his easy bruising tendency. In this age group, one would have to worry whether the patient had leukemia or other blood disease, but the fact that the patient was Jewish, and his grandparents came from Eastern Europe, meaning that he was an Ashkenazi Jew, suggested the diagnosis of Gaucher's disease. This is an inherited metabolic disorder where certain fatty substances accumulate in the liver and spleen and bone marrow. This was proven to be his diagnosis. Fortunately there is effective enzyme therapy to control this genetic error.

In this case the family history was the clue to the diagnosis.

A sixty-four year old man came to the office complaining of left arm pain. He had the pain, on occasion, after he injured the nerve under his left arm while sprinting around a corner when jogging about five years ago. He felt a "rip in my left arm pit." The next two days he had a right hand weakness, diagnosed as a left brachial plexus (nerves coming from the neck to the arm) injury. From that time forward he experienced occasional left arm pain, which suddenly became more frequent the last week before he was seen. Left arm pain can be an indicator of angina, or blocked coronary arteries, but the patient had absolutely no other cardiac symptoms. He attributed the arm pain to a "flare up of the nerve injury." However, his family history did reveal his paternal grandfather to have died of "heart block." Further questioning also revealed that his grandfather's four brothers "all died of heart attacks in their sixties." On the strength of this important family history data a stress test was ordered. The patient failed the test. A coronary artery angiogram demonstrated a major narrowing of his left anterior descending branch of the left coronary artery plus some lesser blocks involving other coronary arteries. He underwent multiple coronary bypass grafts and ten years later he is doing very well.

The family history, in this case, turned our attention away from a brachial plexus injury and toward a cardiac origin.

HABITS

Sleeping

This is an area that your physician should interrogate carefully, for according to the National Institute for Neurological Disorders and Stroke there are forty million people in the U. S. who are afflicted by chronic sleep disorders, and another twenty million who have significant intermittent difficulty falling asleep. It would not be possible to inquire about the seventy sleep disorders that have been classified, but in general they fall into one of three categories: insomnia—lack of sleep; obstructive sleep apnea—seriously disturbed sleep; narcolepsy—excessive sleep; and restless leg syndrome.

Insomnia

Do you have any difficulty falling asleep? Are you unusually tired during the day, and if so is it a disruptive influence in your life? If this is true your physician should determine if there any dietary or emotional factors or environmental factors or stress that could be playing a part in causing your insomnia. On occasion the cause can be a chronic illness, so this line of questioning can be critical.

Obstructive Sleep Apnea

Is your sleep interrupted during the evening? Do you snore? Have you awakened short of breath, or with a rapid pulse, or with severe anxiety? If you answered yes to any of these questions you may be suffering from obstructive sleep apnea, which is the absence of breathing lasting from ten seconds to a minute and caused by a blocked windpipe. The effect is restless and deprived sleep, not to mention the risk for hypertension, heart disease, stroke, diminished mental acuity and the driving risk of falling asleep at the wheel.

If there is a suspicion of a sleep disturbance, a sleep study should be ordered. This is an overnight analysis of your physiological measurements (polysomnograph) while you are asleep.

Narcolepsy

Do you suddenly fall asleep at odd times during the day? This can occur even during activity. This is a genetic disorder usually starting between the ages of fifteen and thirty. Once established, narcolepsy persists throughout life and requires treatment.

Restless Leg Syndrome

Again this is a genetic disorder with unusual tingly leg sensations that causes you to want to keep your legs in motion. Mostly it occurs in the elderly and causes jerking movements that result in insomnia.

Nutrition

The clear-cut correlation between proper nutrition and your health mandates careful evaluation of this part of the history. A physician can obtain a fairly good picture of your nutritional history by asking key questions. How many meals do you eat each day? How many fruits in a day? How many vegetables? In a weeks time how often do you have a high fiber cereal? In a weeks time how often do you eat red meat (beef, pork, lamb, veal)? How many times in a week do you eat fish? What beverages do you usually drink? Do you drink milk? How often do you have desserts or sweets?

By such questioning one can make a determination as to your nutritional intake, and this information could be of critical importance in relationship to your overall medical history.

Exercise

The importance of exercise is well known. It has beneficial cardiovascular effects, it has been reported to delay Alzheimer's disease, it helps maintain proper weight, it acts as an antidepressant, it promotes immune system health and it just plain makes you feel better. The physician should make sure that the amount of exercise you engage in, if any, is evaluated, and depending upon your state of health a proper exercise regimen, where applicable, should be part of your therapeutic program.

Hobbies

A simple question about hobbies will give the physician an idea of who you are. Questions about your personal interests will also demonstrate that the physician is interested in you not only as a medical puzzle to solve, but also as a person with interests and desires.

Tobacco

Since tobacco can cause addiction, cancer of the mouth, tooth decay, gum disease, bad breath, chronic bronchitis, lung cancer, emphysema, elevated blood pressure, elevated pulse rate, accelerated hardening of the arteries, stroke, heart attack, impotence, heartburn, ulcers, pancreatic cancer, bladder cancer and premature death, it is a must that the physician includes this query in your history taking and also offer counseling to stop this deadly habit.

Alcohol

Since alcohol can cause liver disease (hepatitis—cirrhosis—liver failure), gastritis, ulcers, upper gastrointestinal bleeding, cardiac arrhythmias, cardiac enlargement and heart failure, infertility, brain damage, movement disorders, peripheral nerve damage, Parkinson-like symptoms, bone and muscle damage, anemia, acute trauma, and death from any one of the above, it behooves the physician to not only include this query in your history taking exercise, but also to offer counseling to stop this deadly habit. An occasional glass of wine or other alcohol drink is said to impart some cardiac benefit, but anything beyond an occasional alcoholic drink can lead one to the risks outlined above.

Caffeine

Caffeine can cause subtle effects, and the physician should ask you questions related to its use. How much coffee, tea, or soft drinks do you consume in a twenty-four hour period? Caffeine is a central nervous system stimulant and it can cause headaches, insomnia and nervousness. Four or more cups of coffee per day can cause a physical dependence. If you feel a definite need for caffeine then this is enough to assume a degree of addiction. Withdrawal from caffeine can cause fatigue, muscular pain and headache. The effects of too much caffeine on the body can at times be indistinguishable from manic episodes.

CLINICAL EXAMPLES

A forty six year old woman complained of constant fatigue. "Sometimes I have to park in a parking lot and go to sleep for a half hour. When I wake up in the morning I feel like I should be going to bed now." Detailed questioning about her sleep habits prompted the ordering of a sleep study. She was diagnosed as having sleep apnea, but could not tolerate the sleep masks used as treatment. She is still trying, and has seen a dentist who has ordered a dental device designed to aid sleep apnea victims.

An executive of a large company underwent a corporate physical examination. He was found to have an abnormal elevation of three liver enzymes. He came to me in consultation as to the significance of these abnormalities. He was a happily married man with three children and had never received a blood transfusion or had taken illegal drugs. He had an essentially negative history, but the abnormal enzymes prompted questions of alcohol intake. He said he only drank at lunch. "How much?" I asked. "Two a day and none on weekends when I'm home, unless I go out to dinner, then I might have one or two." "What do you drink?" I asked. "Martinis." I told him frankly that physicians have learned to double or triple what a patient tells them if they want to come up with the right amount. He persisted and swore that he never had more than two a day. He would not change his story. I examined him and told him that he did indeed have an enlarged liver. "What does that mean?" he asked. "It could be a fatty liver result-ing from early alcohol liver damage, or cirrhosis from alcohol, or even other liver problems such as hepatitis, but I have to confess two drinks a day shouldn't really cause alcohol liver disease." "How could I find out if alcohol has anything to do with it?" he asked. I told him my recommendation would be to stop drinking 100%, and repeat the tests in two months. If it was from the alcohol the tests should return to normal by then. "Is there a faster way?" he asked. "Yes, a liver biopsy, but I wouldn't recommend it." "Why not?" "Because the procedure is not risk free." "What could happen?" "You could bleed from it, and sometimes that bleeding is life threatening, so the test is not done as cavalierly as drawing a sim-ple blood sample." "I want to have it done," he said. To make a long story short—he insisted, so I referred him to a gastroenterologist and waited to see if the gastroenterologist would agree to perform the biopsy. He did, and the biopsy was positive for alcoholic cirrhosis. Since I only saw him in consultation, the patient went back to his regular physician in an adjacent town. I hope he learned from it and stopped his two drinks a day.

SOCIAL HISTORY

The physician should inquire about your occupation, past and present. Could it have any bearing on your chief complaint and present illness? Are you married, divorced or widowed, and does this status have any relevance to the reason for your visit? Do you have any children? Is your family in good health? Where are you from originally? This type of questioning may or may not have any relationship to your desire for a complete medical examination, but your physician, by showing interest in you, can help enhance the physician-patient relationship.

CLINICAL EXAMPLE

An eighteen year old High School student was brought to the office by his mother. He had lost ten pounds, and "lost all his ambition," according to his mother. I took the young man's history, did a complete physical and found nothing wrong. I told his mother this, and then said I would order tests to be sure of my impression. As the young man looked depressed, I asked his mother if I could speak with her son alone for a while. As it turned out, he was distraught over the loss of a girl friend that "dumped me for another guy." It reminded me of patients I had taken care of who had gone through a bitter divorce. With a number of talk sessions, and an exercise program, the young man resolved the issue, regained his weight and did not require antidepressants.

A middle-aged woman developed a chronic and severe cough. It greatly interfered with her work. She was a speech pathologist and visited clients in their homes. In addition she had a part time job working in a grade school. The cough was so severe her family physician referred her to a lung specialist who diagnosed asthma, or to be more specific—cough variant asthma, and loaded her up with medications and an inhaler. She spoke to me about it, not as a patient, but unofficially, and my only comment was that I couldn't dispute the pulmonologist's diagnosis, but I didn't like the new wording for what physicians, in prior times, called allergic bronchitis. I felt that the asthma title labeled the patient as chronic, and could prevent future health insurance. I did, however, tell her that her mother (a brilliant woman) had a point when she made her own diagnosis. The patient's mother, a retired nurse, had made her own medical observation based upon the patient's social history: "When did the coughing start," the mother asked. "About a year ago," was the reply. "Wasn't that about when you started working at the school?" "Yes, do you think that has something to do with it?" the patient asked. "Maybe—don't you work in one room where you see the kids who come to you for speech problems?" "Yes, I do." "I bet you're allergic to something in that room," the mother said. This was about the time when the patient found it necessary to quit the part-time school job—and sure enough, the cough resolved completely. The summer passed and the patient visited the school room where she had seen the children, and she found the walls completely torn down (as well as the entire wing of the school). She started coughing for the first time in three months, and asked a friend, "What happened here?" "Oh, they had to tear the whole place down," she replied. "How come?" the patient asked. "They found black mold in the walls." There was the answer to the patient's former problem, now completely resolved when she was no longer exposed to the irritating substance—in her case—mold.

This case also illustrates the fact that a well trained nurse can take an excellent history and a well trained physician can miss important facts!

All the more reason to take charge of your health and always seek answers.

SYSTEM REVIEW

Introduction

A careful review of the various organ systems is included in this section of the medical history. The purpose of the system review is to search for symptoms other than may have so far been elicited in the taking of the biographical data, chief complaint, present history, past history, family history, habits and social history. The system review is important in order to determine if there are any symptoms involving other parts of your body that may be related to the chief complaint and present illness, or may represent new clues suggesting other organ system problems. It is no surprise that critically important information surfaces at this point. The physician may choose to ask you these questions separately during the taking of the history, or may ask the questions while performing the physical examination of the organ system. Only positive and pertinent negative responses are documented in this part of the medical history. This is reminiscent of a computerized medical history, which can be programmed to record the positive and pertinent negative responses entered by the patient. Your physician will uncover information during the system review query that he may not be equipped to handle, but this information, which may be crucial to your well being, will enable the doctor to refer you to the appropriate specialist.

I will go through each organ system and ask the questions that a physician should ask in order to assist in capturing important medical history information.

Skin (including hair and nails)

Have you had any previous skin problem? Do you have any birthmarks? Have you ever been tattooed? The last question about tattoos may have relevance if your physician is suspecting you of having hepatitis (unsterile tattoo needle).

Do you have a sore that is healing poorly? Have you noticed any unusual growths on your skin? Have you noticed any black or brown streaks under your nails? Do you have any hard, firm skin lesions? Have you noted any moles or skin spots that are asymmetrical, have an irregular border, have exhibited a color change, have increased in size, developed scaling, flaking, or oozing, began to itch, developed tenderness, or have you developed a redness surrounding a mole? Any one of these questions, if answered positively, should raise the suspicion of a malignant skin lesion such as a squamous cell carcinoma, basal cell carcinoma, or a malignant melanoma. The last diagnosis has the most serious connotations.

The skin is the mirror of the body and much about internal pathology can be learned by careful evaluation of the skin.

Have you had any increased pigmentation (darkening) of the skin?

If localized, this may represent vitiligo, a loss of pigmentation that causes lighter skin patches in sharp contrast to the normal skin that appears darker. If the loss of pigment is generalized, this can be seen in chronic kidney disease and hyper or hypothyroidism. A Caucasian who develops Addison's disease (adrenal gland failure) will develop a significant tanning effect. An African-American who gets Addison's will literally turn pitch black. Other causes of increased pigmentation of the skin includes cirrhosis of the liver or hemochromatosis, which is a familial or acquired disorder where iron gets deposited in the skin and other organs. Increased pigmentation of the skin may occur normally during pregnancy.

Do you have any unusual itching of the skin?

Itching (pruritis) of the skin can be seen in chronic kidney disease. It can also occur with the rash of vasculitis (inflammation of blood vessels). This could be a clue to an autoimmune disorder where your immune system rejects parts of your body. Other causes of itching include yellow jaundice resulting from liver disease and/or obstructive disease of the gall bladder and liver bile ducts caused by gallstones or pancreatic malignancy. Other internal malignancies can also cause skin itching.

Has your skin been excessively dry?

Excessive dryness (xerosis) can be seen in chronic kidney disease and hypothyroidism (underactive thyroid gland).

These are just a few of the examples of the kind of information that one can get from a careful skin system review.

Have you had any nail changes? If the answer is yes, more specific questioning should follow. The question about nail changes will prompt you to look at your nails. Important clues to a diagnosis can come from changes, such as pits, ridges, thickening, streaks and color changes. Pits, ridges or thickening can be seen in iron deficiency anemia, fungal infections of the nails and psoriasis. Pigmented streaks can be seen in Addison's disease. Prominent bulging nails called clubbing are seen in lung diseases. Various drugs can result in nail color changes: tetracycline antibiotic (yellow) and antimalarial drugs (blue). The pseudomonas bacteria can cause green nails.

If you complain of hair loss reflected by small patches of hair that have fallen out, you are suffering from alopecia (partial spotty baldness). The cause is more often than not unknown, but it can be a clue to an underactive thyroid gland, an underactive pituitary gland, early syphilis, stress, reaction to hair chemicals, toxicity from some drugs and overdose of vitamin A.

Thinning hair, mostly caused by genetic predisposition, can at times be the clue to an over or underactive thyroid gland, chemotherapy, hormone replacement medications such as birth control pills and environmental toxins.

CLINICAL EXAMPLES

Four members of an African American family visited the dermatology clinic at Cook County Hospital—a man, his wife, and two teen aged children. The husband of the patient stated that he brought his wife because "her skin was getting darker and darker." Indeed, the patient's husband and the two children were relatively light skinned, in sharp contrast to the wife and mother. The patient also complained of severe fatigue, and her blood pressure was 90/56. The diagnosis of Addison's disease, an autoimmune gradual self destruction of the adrenal glands, was easily established and the patient was started on cortisone replacement therapy.

A thirty-seven year old man presented with a single symptom of diffuse itching. A complete medical history and physical examination was unremarkable except for some signs of skin irritation induced by the patient's intense scratching. He was treated symptomatically and supportively and had some partial relief, but the symptoms would remit and exacerbate. After about a year of this he developed a neck mass, biopsy of which was determined to be Hodgkin's disease. This is a lymph gland malignancy with a good prognosis if caught early. With therapy for his underlying disease the patient's itching stopped. In this case the cause of the itching could not be determined until the patient had developed enlarged lymph nodes.

Breast

Do you perform breast self-examination? Most patients answer no to this question. Breast self examinations have been taught and advocated for many years, but a recent study of 200,000 women in China failed to show that these exams reduced deaths from breast cancer. I have nothing against this exam as long as women think of it as a means of getting to know what their normal breast looks and feels like, so that a sudden change will be recognized, and understand that the self examination is a screening test third in importance to regular screening mammography and careful physician examination.

The mammogram exam is the only screening method that has proven to be effective in reducing breast cancer deaths. It is effective in detecting cancer at an early stage when the cancer is too small to be picked up by self-examination and professional examination. Mammography can pick up lumps the size of a pencil eraser whereas the self and physician examination will ordinarily require a lesion about a size of a nickel, assuming a thin breast. Obesity mitigates against the effectiveness of self or physician examination.

Other questions that should be asked are:
Do you have any breast pain?
If the answer is yes, the reason needs to be investigated carefully. It is less likely that the cause is cancer because a malignancy of the breast usually is not accompanied by pain, although about ten percent of women do describe a vague type of pain as the first indication of cancer of the breast. The pain is usually not severe, but rather described as burning or pulling.

The most common cause of pain is the effect of estrogen and progesterone hormones during the second half of the menstrual cycle. This effect is worse before a menstrual period and gets better with menstruation. The effect of these hormones is to cause the breast to become tender and lumpy. Caffeine has a chemical called methylxanthine that causes blood vessels to dilate resulting in further distention of the breast causing more pain. High salt diets that cause fluid retention can also enhance this effect.

Antidepressant medications and stress may also cause breast pain.

A bacterial infection is suggested when there is a localized breast pain, redness and tenderness.

A second question is: are your breasts lumpy, or have your breasts gotten lumpier lately?

This problem is called fibrocystic disease. Other names are benign breast disease or mammary dysplasia. The condition usually disappears after menopause unless the woman is taking hormone replacement therapy. As mentioned above, caffeine should be avoided.

Have you experienced nipple discharge from one or both breasts?

This is the third most common breast complaint behind lumpiness and pain. A nipple discharge should raise concern if it appears without squeezing the nipple, if it is bloody, if it is black or brown in color, if it is sticky, if it is clear (unlike breast milk) and if it is one sided.

If the discharge meets any of these criteria a search for a cause is a must. These include a pituitary tumor that liberates excess prolactin hormone. This hormone is responsible for breast gland growth that results in milk production. In the case of a pituitary tumor the discharge will involve both breasts.

Bloody or watery secretions are mostly caused by a benign papilloma (a wart-like tumor that grows inside of a milk duct). This problem usually involves only one breast.

Other causes of nipple discharge are fibrocystic disease, and widening and hardening of the ducts common in the elderly. Also a clear nipple discharge may be caused by medications such as birth control pills, digitalis, diuretics, cortisone and tricyclic antidepressants.

Not to be forgotten is nipple discharge in men. In puberty the discharge is not unusual and of no clinical significance. In the adult male, however, a discharge is frequently associated with cancer, and mammography and biopsy should be performed.

CLINICAL EXAMPLES

A twenty-four year old female graduate student complained of sudden onset of bilateral milky nipple discharge. She was unmarried and had not missed any menstrual periods. Bilateral nipple discharge is called galactorrhea and is due to increased prolactin hormone production from the pituitary gland. She had no other symptoms. She often "smoked a joint" with some friends. She went on the internet and did a Google search where she found that nipple discharge, if bilateral, is called galactorrhea. She did another Google search for galactorrhea, and found a list of the causes—one of which was marijuana. She stopped the marijuana, and the nipple discharge disappeared. In this case, she took charge of her health very well—belatedly.

A fifty-four year old woman complained of a one month history of a rust-colored nipple discharge from the right breast. Physical examination revealed only some mild tenderness, but no palpable mass. A mammogram was negative, but the possibility of the patient having an early malignancy was good. As best as could be ascertained it appeared that the discharge was coming from one duct. She was referred to a surgeon who operated on the patient. She had a carcinoma-in-situ, which is a very early cancer involving only the cell lining of the duct. Her prognosis is excellent.

Eyes

Primary care physicians can do little to treat serious eye problems. They have not been trained in the use of complicated eye instruments. They can, however, ask some simple questions that can lead to the possibility of eye problems urgently in need of evaluation.

Do you have any eye pain?

If the answer is yes your physician can evaluate whether or not you have a clearly visible local reason such as a treatable eye infection (conjunctivitis). If not, he will have to determine if the eye complaint may be part of your chief complaint and present illness. If there is doubt about this possibility, then you will need referral to an ophthalmologist, especially if the reason for your eye pain is not obvious on your physician's screening examination. Sixty-five reasons for eye pain have been documented, and pinning it down may be beyond your primary care physician's capability.

Do you have any changes in your vision?

If there is a positive response to this question your physician will need to differentiate between the various types of visual loss or change. These include blindness, partial vision loss or distortion, night blindness, impaired vision, cloudy vision, double vision, blind spot, central visual loss and peripheral visual loss. Well over 100 causes for these problems local to the eye, or representing medical, traumatic, or surgical problems have been identified. Needless to say, an ophthalmology referral is necessary.

CLINICAL EXAMPLES

A sixty-nine year old male came to the office complaining that "I got blind in one eye. It was like a curtain came over it. It only lasted about a minute." This is a classical description of amaurosis fugax. Amaurosis from the Greek meaning dark, and fugax from the latin meaning fleeting. This strongly suggests a vascular cause, but there are other causes, including eye diseases, migraine and other miscellaneous diseases. The main cause is a stroke until proven otherwise, so this prompted an evaluation of the blood vessels to the brain. In this patient's case there were no major blood vessel blockages, there were no abnormalities on the neurological or eye examination, and there was no history of migraine. The presumptive diagnosis was a transient ischemic cerebral attack, meaning a temporary blockage of an artery to the brain due to spasm or clot.

A seventy-two year old woman came to the office with multiple complaints, one of which was eye pain. She was given a complete examination including a cursory eye exam. One of the more common causes of eye pain is glaucoma. If untreated, it can lead to blindness. In glaucoma, the interior eye fluid is under increased pressure. This can be easily measured with the proper instrument that is not usually available in a primary care physician's office. A rough estimate of the pressure can be made by having the patient close her eyes. The doctor then touches the closed eyelids with the tip of the second and middle finger and gently presses on the eyeball. Normally the eyeballs are soft and give a little under the pressing finger. With glaucoma the increased pressure causes the eyeballs to be more rigid, and this was the impression I got. That is only presumptive evidence, however, but glaucoma was confirmed in the ophthalmologist's office. In the majority of cases it is easily treatable with eye drops.

Ears

Have you noticed any hearing loss?

If the response is yes, your physician needs to consider the possibilities. Hearing loss is divided into two types:

The first is conductive hearing loss—an interference with the transmission of sound from the outer to the inner ear. The causes are numerous and range from ear infections to fluid in the inner ear to ear canal blockage from wax. Your physician can help you with these problems. Other causes of conductive hearing loss will require the services of an ear specialist.

The second type of hearing loss is called sensorineural hearing loss, caused by disruption of the pathway for sound impulses from the inner ear through the auditory nerve and to the brain. This is more serious, but there are some reversible causes such as hearing loss from certain drugs such as aspirin, quinine and some antibiotics. A careful evaluation by an ear specialist or neurologist is necessary to uncover the more serious causes, which range from age related hearing loss to tumors, viral infection, stroke and multiple sclerosis.

Any sudden hearing loss in one or both ears, especially in the absence of an upper respiratory infection, should require a referral to an ear specialist.

Have you experienced a sensation of spinning or whirling? This is a sensation of movement and is known as subjective vertigo. A similar question would be: do objects spin around you? This is known as objective vertigo. It is not enough to ask, are you dizzy? This answer to this question will depend upon your interpretation of the word dizzy, which may be defined as light-headedness, a feeling of fainting, or unsteadiness. These three interpretations may carry with it multiple different connotations as to diagnosis in the mind of the physician.

Vertigo is not a diagnosis. It is a symptom due to many different diagnoses. In reference to the ear, vertigo results from a disturbance of the vestibular system, a system involving the inner ear, the vestibular nerve and the brain. They work together and are responsible for keeping objects in visual focus regardless of how the body moves.

Your physician may be able to identify a cause of vertigo, including an inner ear infection (otitis media), certain antibiotics, quinine, aspirin, some over the counter cold medicines, some chemotherapy agents, alcohol, diuretics, antidepressants, anticonvulsants and exposure to lead or mercury. Other causes may require consultation from a neurologist.

CLINICAL EXAMPLES

A seventy-six year old man came to the office in a follow-up visit for his hypertension. Before he left he mentioned that "My wife will be mad if I don't tell you that she thinks I'm getting deaf." He then told of the arguments between the two of them, accusing each other of not being able to hear. He no longer watches TV with her because when he turns up the volume his wife says, "The walls are shaking," and she leaves the room, or she'll say "thank God we don't live in an apartment anymore because the neighbors would be banging on the walls." I took a quick view of his ear canals and did not see any significant obstructing wax, and the ear drums looked okay. But an audiologist confirmed his wife's clinical impression. He was fitted for hearing aids. Harmony has now returned to the household.

A thirty-nine year old woman came to my office for a complete physical examination. She had stopped in a drug store and took her blood pressure on an automated machine. When she found it to be elevated, she repeated the BP check on two more occasions, and the reading remained essentially the same. During the medical history it was learned that on several occasions, she had three or four bouts of "dizziness," became "unsteady on my feet" and "heard a roaring in my ears." These attacks would last about a day and then stop. After her third attack she wondered if her blood pressure was elevated, and that was the reason for her drug store visits. The physical examination did reveal a blood pressure of 160/90, but her symptoms did not exactly fit a diagnosis of high blood pressure. I asked her to describe what she meant by dizziness and her description was more classically vertigo. Her ear examination was entirely normal, but some office based ear tests raised the possibility of a slight hearing loss. I ordered basic screening laboratory studies, and they eventually came back within normal limits. I started her on a diuretic for her elevated blood pressure and sent her to an ear specialist. Luck was with me for the specialist diagnosed Meniere's syndrome, an inner ear disorder characterized by vertigo, hearing loss and tinnitus, and, as it turned out, the diuretic I ordered was also recommended by the ENT specialist as therapy for her Meniere's syndrome. The condition is not curable, but it is controllable.

Nose

Do you have nasal drainage or obstruction? If the problem is of a chronic nature, then the causes include allergies, nasal spray overuse, sinusitis, and some medications such as birth control pills. There are also local causes such as nasal polyps, deviated nasal septum, and large adenoids (lymph tissue in the back of the throat).

Have you had any nosebleeds (epistaxis)? Here again the causes are numerous and could range from a hot and dry climate where the nasal lining may crack causing bleeding, to upper respiratory infection, allergies and exposure to chemicals. There are also medical conditions that present with a nosebleed as its initial symptom. These include kidney failure and low levels of blood platelets needed for clotting. Blood platelets can be reduced by unknown reasons, by toxins, medications and as part of blood diseases such as leukemia. Increased alcohol use may interfere with normal platelet production and result in nosebleeds as well. Medications such as aspirin and ibuprofen (motrin and advil) can also cause nosebleeds.

CLINICAL EXAMPLES

A fifty-two year old Chinese man came to the office with complaints of progressively increasing right-sided nasal blockage and occasional bloody nasal drainage. Examination revealed only two hard and firm lymph glands on both sides of the upper neck. An examination of his exterior nasal passages was unrevealing. He was sent to an ear, nose, and throat specialist who confirmed the diagnosis of nasopharyngeal carcinoma, not an uncommon malignancy in people of Chinese ancestry.

A patient came to my office for a complete medical examination. The chief complaint was gastrointestinal in nature. In taking a system review the patient stated that he had nasal congestion for years, but "I live with it." Examination of his nose revealed that he had what looked like many 'seedless grapes' that indeed were obstructing his nasal passageway. He was diagnosed with nasal polyps, an allergic condition. He was sent to an ear, nose and throat specialist, and the polyps were removed surgically, affording him substantial relief.

This case demonstrates that a carefully taken system review can elicit problems not related to the patient's chief complaint, and afford the patient considerable relief.

Mouth

Like the skin, mouth symptoms may be a reflection of local or generalized disease. Do you have a sore or painful mouth? This is a critical first question. If yes, the local causes may include braces, a poorly fitting denture, a sharp or broken tooth and chewing tobacco.

An infection may cause a painful mouth. The causes include a herpes virus, which can lie dormant in the body for many years and manifest itself during the course of an illness or fever or stress. A yeast infection (thrush) caused by a yeast known as candida albicans is a relatively important cause of a sore mouth. In adults, thrush occurs in diabetics, during the course of taking steroids (cortisone) and immunosuppresive (chemotherapy) agents that suppress the immune system, or in conditions where the immune system is already suppressed such as HIV-

AIDS. As illustrated before, a thrush infection of the mouth may be the first sign of AIDS.

Do you have any lumps in your mouth? A positive response should elicit a careful search for cancer, or less serious problems such as benign cysts to torus mandibularis or torus palaltinus, a benign bony overgrowth on the inside of the jaw or hard palate.

Do you have any abnormal taste in your mouth? This may be caused by dental infections, salivary gland infections, or gastro-esophageal reflux disease where acid or bile in the stomach refluxes (goes back up the esophagus) to your mouth.

CLINICAL EXAMPLES

A fifty-two year old woman was seen in my office with a chief complaint of fatigue and joint pains. The system review did elicit the fact that her "mouth was always dry and I carry a water bottle with me wherever I go." A diagnosis of Sjogren's syndrome was made on the basis of the symptoms described. It was confirmed. This is an autoimmune inflammatory disorder, characterized by dry mouth, dry eyes, arthritis, plus a long list of other possible symptoms. The disease is chronic and treated symptomatically, but the patient was at least relieved to discover that she "wasn't a neurotic after all."

A young man came to the emergency room of Cook County hospital in severe distress. He was holding his neck and jaw with his right hand. His facial expression was distorted into a grimace clearly exemplifying the agony he was experiencing. When asked what was wrong, he could only continue holding his neck, and with the index finger of his left hand pointed to his throat. He had difficulty opening his mouth, but I did manage to get an adequate look and discovered a large peritonsillar abscess on the right. The normal anatomy was completely distorted by this large puss filled mass which almost extended to the other side obstructing his throat. This is a severe and thankfully rare complication of a sore throat gone unattended, but there is nothing so gratifying to the patient (and doctor) as to see the immediate relief that ensues when an incision is made in this pus-filled pocket and the pus literally spouts out and a smile comes over the relieved patient's face.

Throat

Do you have a sore throat? The most common cause is a viral or bacterial infection. A throat culture may need to be done in order to determine if the problem is due to the strep germ, which if untreated can result in serious cardiac or kidney problems. Gastroesophageal reflux disease (GERD) where stomach acid regurgitates into the mouth may also cause a sore throat.

Is your voice hoarse? If you are a smoker, and if the hoarseness has persisted for more than six weeks, laryngeal cancer (cancer of the voice box) must be considered. Less serious causes of hoarseness include voice strain, benign vocal cord polyps, an upper respiratory infection and gastroesophageal reflux.

The good news is that for non-smokers, oral, throat, laryngeal, or head and neck cancer is very rare, but if you are a smoker and have any of the following symptoms you should not hesitate to seek medical care:

1. A voice hoarseness lasting more than six weeks.

2. A sore throat lasting more than two weeks.

3. Difficulty swallowing food in the absence of or presence of sore throat pain that lasts more than two weeks.

4. Sudden unexplained weight loss.

5. A neck lump persisting for more than two weeks.

6. A non-healing mouth sore or ulcer.

CLINICAL EXAMPLES

An elderly female was seen in my office for fatigue and bilateral knee pain severely limiting her ability to walk. In taking the medical history it was apparent to me that her voice was very hoarse. "Oh, no, I always talk that way," she said. "Do you smoke?" I asked. "Yes," she responded. Both she and her husband had smoked for sixty years. I asked her husband and daughter if they didn't think the patient's voice was hoarse. They assured me that "that's the way she's always talked," and seemed a little irritated that I was zeroing in on an unimportant issue not related to the purpose of her visit. Seeing their response, I concentrated on the patient's chief complaints, but when they left, I did recommend that they see an ear nose and throat specialist just to be sure there was no problem with her vocal cords, because there was always a possibility that a very slowly evolving hoarseness (a possible symptom of vocal cord pathology) could be missed by loved ones who hear her talking very day. They did see the specialist who found several polyps on her vocal cords. They were removed surgically. Fortunately they were benign. Neither she nor her husband has stopped smoking.

This is another example of where information not related to the chief complaint and picked up during the system review resulted in significant information.

A nineteen year old young man came to my office complaining of severe sore throat, fever and fatigue. In looking in his throat, I found petechiae at the junction of his hard and soft palate. Petechiae are small reddish or purplish spots caused by minute hemorrhages. This is classical for infectious mononucleosis, which was confirmed by a complete blood count and a blood test known as the heterophile antibody test. This is a viral disease and time and rest are curative.

Cardiovascular

Do you have a past history of elevated cholesterol or triglyceride? Have you ever been told that you have a heart murmur, congenital heart disease, rheumatic heart disease, or hypertension? How far can you walk? These questions will give your physician a quick insight to any past history of a cardiac problem as well as your exercise ability, which provides a good clue as to your overall cardiac status.

Do you have any chest pain or tightness? A yes response should elicit the list of questions we already went through in evaluating the chief complaint. The purpose is to determine if the pain complaint is typically cardiac or may represent another problem. This is a critical issue upon which depends the proper diagnosis.

Do you have any missed heartbeats, or "skipped beats," or absent beats? This is a common symptom experienced by most people at one time or another. If you are young and healthy these may be of no clinical significance. These beats may be caused or worsened by caffeine in coffee, tea, or cola drinks, and by alcohol and some cold, hay fever and asthma medications.

They should, however, be investigated if:

1. Your "skipped beats" are frequent and bothersome enough to disrupt your life.

2. You are middle aged or elderly.

3. You have known risk factors for cardiac disease.

4. You have a known history of a cardiac problem.

5. Your "skipped beats" are associated with dizziness, lightheadedness, or loss of consciousness.

If you fall in any of the above categories, your physician will order an electro-cardiogram or a twenty-four hour holter monitor, which records your heartbeat for a full day. In the event that neither of these tests capture the "skipped beats," an event recorder can be used. This device uses a circular tape that can record thirty seconds of your heart rhythm. When you experience the skipped beats, or other symptom of concern, you press a button that freezes the recording, which is then transmitted over telephone lines to the interpreter. The event recorder can be used for an extended period of time (two months).

Have you ever experienced a rapid and regular heartbeat (tachycardia)?

Tachycardia is defined as any regular heartbeat over 100 beats per minute in a resting adult. A persistent tachycardia can be harmful, as a rapidly beating heart does not perform efficiently. First, there is not enough time for the ventricles to fill completely causing the blood output from the heart to the rest of the body to decrease. Second, the heart workload increases causing it to need more oxygen. In a young, healthy person this may be of little consequence, but in one with a history of a cardiac problem this could result in a significant oxygen lack causing damage or death of heart muscle (heart attack).

The term tachycardia simply means fast heartbeat, and its causes can be external to the heart such as with an overactive thyroid gland or an autonomic nervous system dysfunction. Or the cause of tachycardia may be related to the hearts electrical system. There are three cardiac electrical disturbances:

1. If the heart's electrical system is working normally, and if the rate is over 100 beats per minute to 150 beats per minute, then this is called sinus tachycardia. There may be normal physiology at play here or it may have an endocrine (hyperthyroidism) or autonomic nervous system etiology.

2.   If the hearts electrical system is working abnormally there are two possible causes of a rapid, regular heartbeat. First, when the abnormal electrical impulse originates in the atria, the chambers above the ventricles of the heart, it takes a circular route and beats more than 150 beats per minute. This heart rate, originating in the atria, is called supraventricular tachycardia, meaning above the ventricles. If the ventricles beat this fast it is known as ventricular tachycardia. This latter rapid heart rate in an already damaged heart, if it persists, carries with it serious implications including ventricular fibrillation, which is a fluttering of the ventricles resulting in stoppage of the flow of blood and death.

Your physician must carefully evaluate the information you give him about a rapid and regular heartbeat. Its cause must be identified exactly so therapy, if proven necessary, is started promptly.

Have you experienced any shortness of breath? Do you wheeze? Do you cough? Have you awakened from a sound sleep gasping for breath? Do you have difficult sleeping flat without pillows because it results in shortness of breath? Are you extremely tired?

All these questions are geared to give your physician a clue to the possibility that you are experiencing left ventricular heart failure. Your failing left ventricle is causing congestion and increased pressure of blood in the veins of your lungs causing fluid to back up in your lungs.

Do you have swelling of the legs or abdomen?

There are numerous causes of these symptoms, but one of them may be right ventricular heart failure casing pressure to increase in the veins of your body resulting in fluid leakage in your legs and abdomen. This may be due to other causes but should raise the suspicion of right ventricular heart failure until proven otherwise.

Should you manifest any of these symptoms, your physician must search for a cardiac reason. These include:

1.   High blood pressure causing a strain and enlargement of your heart.

2.   Blocked heart arteries causing damage or death of heart muscle.

3.   Heart valve diseases causing a strain on the various chambers of the heart.

4. Cardiomyopathy—a chronic disease of the heart muscle.

5. Congenital heart disease.

6. Extra cardiac causes including severe anemia (rare), decreased metabolism from an underactive thyroid, or increased metabolism from an overactive thyroid (rare) and liver or kidney failure.

Heart failure can be progressive, but proper diagnosis and treatment can either eliminate the cause or slow the progression and improve quality of life.

Do you have pains in your legs, hip or back when you walk that is relieved when you rest?

If you answer yes to this query you may be suffering from intermittent claudication (pain due to decreased circulation to your legs resulting from a blocked artery or arteries). This is a symptom of peripheral artery disease. In intermittent claudication your blood flow to your legs are sufficient at rest, but when you walk, the artery blockage prevents the muscles from getting the increased blood necessary to meet the demands of exercise. This results in pain when walking. The symptom is clear-cut and diagnostic, and if severe enough should alert your physician to performing the necessary confirming tests.

CLINICAL EXAMPLES

When I was in medical school, one of my professors told us about a patient who he saw in consultation. This middle aged man was in chronic heart failure. In those days all that was available for heart failure was a toxic mercury-based diuretic (mercuhydrin), digitalis and a very low salt diet. This was also the days before cardiac surgery. The long-term prognosis for patients with this diagnosis was poor—they were usually not expected to live more than two years. Nowadays, of course, there is very effective life prolonging therapy for this condition. After the patient was seen, and my professor made what recommendations he could, the patient thanked him and said, "Well, now back to the salt mines." The professor laughed, thinking he meant he was going back to work, but he managed to ask, "Oh, what kind of work do you do?" "I work in the salt mines," the patient said. If I remember correctly, this took place in Minnesota. This bit of social history could have been very important in this patient's therapy. There he was, working in a salt mine, eating lunch with salt falling all over his food etc. According to the professor, after he was urged to stop working in the salt mines, his condition improved greatly and he was well controlled on digitalis alone.

A sixty-six year old man came under my care for advanced arteriosclerotic heart disease. He had severe angina and took a beta blocker and nitroglycerin. When I first saw him, he was on the maximum dose of the beta blocker, and his condition was so advanced that he had chest pain on walking and had to be brought into the office in a wheel chair. In fact, when I would ask him to get up on the examining table from his chair, he would have to put a nitroglycerin tablet under his tongue to prevent the cardiac pain that would invariably occur just from walking the few feet to the examining table and sitting down. This patient was seen during the early days of cardiac surgery when there were very few medications for this condition, so I felt that the new surgical approach could be an option for this severely disabled patient. I sent him to the local university center, and they did a coronary artery angiogram and declared him inoperable. Not dissuaded, I referred him to one of my medical school classmates, a pioneer in cardiac surgery—Dr. Dudley Johnson of Milwaukee, Wisconsin. Dudley saw him and operated. He did, if my memory serves me correctly, seven bypasses. I saw the patient six weeks later. He was not brought in a wheel chair, but rather walked in briskly to the office. In fact he said, "Watch me, doc," and promptly took off on a brisk walk up and down my office corridor. This gentleman was a widower, and he surprised me with his next request. "I've got a favor to ask, doc." "What's that?" I asked. "I want you to send me to a urologist." "Oh, what's wrong?" I asked. "Nothing—I want to get a penile implant." Taken aback, I said, "But, you just had major heart surgery." After further thinking about the miracle wrought by Dudley, I also said, "Don't tell me you've got a girl friend already!" "No," he said, "but I'm going to get one."

Pulmonary

Queries in the pulmonary system will be geared to attempt to determine the type of lung problem, if any, you may have. Do you have shortness of breath? Do you have wheezing? Do you awaken at night short of breath? The state of your pulmonary or cardiac status can be determined by these questions.

Do you cough? How do you describe your cough? Is it dry or productive of sputum? How often do you cough? If it is throughout the entire day you may have an upper respiratory infection. If you only cough during certain times of the day, does it represent exposure to irritants such as mold or other environmental triggers? Do you only cough at night? If so, you may have sinusitis or a postnasal drip. When you cough do you bring up sputum? Is the sputum colored? If so, this may be a bacterial infection and you may need antibiotics and follow up care.

Have you coughed up blood? This is an important symptom and raises the possibility of many disorders: trauma, infections of many types, cancer and bronchial disorders. World wide, tuberculosis is the most common reason for coughing up blood (hemoptysis). The cause of hemoptysis must be identified.

The answer to any one of these questions should also alert the physician to one of the three basic types of lung disorder that interferes with normal lung function:

The first is obstructive lung disease. The most common causes in this category are asthma, chronic bronchitis and emphysema. The pathology here is a narrowing or blockage of the airways that result in decreased exhaled air flow.

The second is restrictive lung diseases, which decreases the amount of air that your lungs can hold. This results from a decrease in the lung's elasticity or impaired chest wall expansion during inhalation. Examples here include occupational illnesses such as asbestosis, and pulmonary fibrosis (scarring of the lungs).

The third type is known as defective lung disease where the air is unable to easily get from the air sacs to the blood.

Most lung problems usually involve a combination of these pathological mechanisms. Any suspicion should alert your physician to various pulmonary function tests that can differentiate between the types of lung problem you may have.

CLINICAL EXAMPLES

A middle-aged woman was under my care for vitamin B12 deficiency resulting in a severe anemia. She also had hypothyroidism. She was diagnosed three years prior, had been placed on therapy and was well controlled. I saw her every six months in follow up. These two problems are autoimmune illnesses. In the first instance the body fails to absorb B12, resulting in decreased and abnormal blood production, and in the second instance the thyroid gland fails to make an adequate supply of thyroid hormone. By providing the patient with monthly B12 injections and oral thyroid hormone replacement, the patient is well—not cured—but well. If one has to come down with an autoimmune disease, one of these should be chosen. But as is often the case, if a patient has one autoimmune disease, they can be prone to getting another. That's why I was very worried when I received a call from her telling me that she had developed shortness of breath, and wanted to see me right away. When she came to the office her examination was essentially unchanged from previous exams with the exception of perhaps some decreased breath sounds, but I felt that a chest X-ray was indicated. It revealed a condition called pulmonary fibrosis, also known as interstitial lung disease. This is almost certainly an autoimmune disease where the lung slowly scars over, but it is nowhere near as amenable to therapy as the other two. She was eventually started on cortisone, which gave her symptomatic relief, but unfortunately she experienced a slowly progressive downhill course.

A sixty-two year old physician became short of breath. He was examined and discovered to have a loud cardiac murmur. He denied ever having been made aware of this before. A chest X-ray was ordered and demonstrated a large mediastinal tumor. This is a tumor located in the center of the chest in front of the heart. Apparently the tumor put pressure on the heart, caused the murmur and compromised cardiac function. Surgical biopsy proved the tumor to be a thymosarcoma, an extremely rare and malignant tumor of the thymus gland. The thymus gland is important in immunity, is prominent at birth, and shrinks down as one gets older. In the long history of the Mayo Clinic (at that time—about twenty years ago) they had seventeen cases in their registry.

Gastrointestinal

The gastrointestinal system stretches from the mouth through the pharynx, down the esophagus, into the stomach, through the small intestine (about twenty-two feet), through the large intestine (ascending, transverse and descending colon), and through the rectum and anus. Also included are the liver, the gall bladder and its ducts into the intestine and the pancreas and its duct. Needless to say the symptoms involving such a lengthy and complicated multi-functional system are numerous, but your physician must try to ask those questions which should give vital information concerning the functioning of your gastrointestinal system. The questioning is complicated by the fact that many of the symptoms attributed to the gastrointestinal tract may be caused by other body systems. Your physician must carefully sort this out.

Do you have any abdominal pain? Is it diffuse or localized?
If either one, details must be sought. The abdomen is divided up into four quadrants, so the exact location of the pain is important to help pin point the abdominal organ involved. For example: right upper quadrant (liver or gallblad-

der); left upper quadrant (stomach or pancreas or spleen); right lower quadrant (appendix); left lower quadrant (descending colon); pit of the stomach or upper center (stomach, small intestine, gallbladder, pancreas).

Have you had an increase in your abdominal girth? This may be due to simple weight gain, or it may represent fluid in the belly (ascites) as a result of liver failure or heart failure. Increased abdominal girth due to gas may be due to intestinal distention secondary to irritable bowel (spastic colitis). An intestinal obstruction, which could increase your abdominal girth will usually present very suddenly and be associated with severe pain, nausea and vomiting.

Do you suffer from constipation—the difficult passage of hard stools? If the answer is yes, it may be due to simple causes such as dehydration, the absence of dietary fiber in your diet, certain diuretic medications, or medicines containing iron or calcium. More serious causes, which slow intestinal transit time, include a low potassium level, underactive thyroid gland, other severe illnesses and medications such as codeine, morphine and antidepressants. Bowel blockage caused by infection, strictures or tumors are also important causes of constipation.

Do you have diarrhea? We all do at one time or another and mostly the causes are dietary, or are related to transient infections by a virus or bacteria. If, however, the symptoms persist and are accompanied by abdominal cramps, pain, fever, or bleeding, an investigative evaluation is warranted to rule out chronic illnesses such as ileitis or Crohn's disease, autoimmune inflammations of the gastrointestinal tract.

Do you have black stools (melena)—black like tar or coal? This symptom is associated with upper gastrointestinal hemorrhage. As the blood passes from the upper gastrointestinal tract through the small intestine and colon, the iron in the blood is oxidized and turns black. A search for upper gastrointestinal bleeding, particularly the esophagus, stomach or duodenum (first part of the small intestine), must be undertaken on an urgent basis. Causes include peptic ulcers, polyps, esophageal varices (dilated veins), esophageal tears, inflamed stomach (gastritis) and cancer.

Have you passed bright red blood with a bowel movement? This symptom indicates that you are bleeding from a lower intestinal source such as the upper colon, sigmoid colon and rectum. The blood acts as a cathartic, which results in a prompt passage out of the body. The first thoughts are hemorrhoids (dilated anal veins), diverticulosis (colon pockets), inflammatory bowel disease, polyps, or cancer. A search for a definite cause is mandatory.

Do you complain of dyspepsia? This should be defined to you as abdominal pain or discomfort, usually in the pit of the stomach, constant or episodic, and, at times, may be associated with nausea or vomiting, bloating, heartburn, or belching. This is probably the most common gastrointestinal complaint, occurring in as many as forty percent of patients. The causes are numerous and range from a "nervous stomach," to peptic ulcer disease, gallbladder disease, gastroesophageal reflux disease, gastritis, pancreatitis, or cancer.

Have you ever experienced yellow jaundice (yellow skin and eyes)?
This occurs when your blood carries an excess of the pigment known as bilirubin, which arises from the normal breakdown of red blood cells in your body. The bilirubin is excreted by the liver into the bile. If the liver is not working well, or the liver or gall bladder ducts are blocked (so the bile cannot enter your intestines) then the bile backs up in the blood stream and gets deposited in your skin turning it yellow. The cause of yellow jaundice must be thoroughly investigated so that treatment will be instituted promptly. The causes include: excess breakdown of red blood cells (hemolysis) that has exceeded the liver's capacity to handle the increased bilirubin; Hemolysis can be caused by some medications; Jaundice can be caused by hepatitis due to viral infection of the liver, or scarring of the liver (cirrhosis) from alcohol or viruses; Gallbladder stones can block ducts that will prevent the bilirubin from being excreted in the intestines and can result in jaundice; Pancreatic cancer can do the same.
Jaundice is an important symptom demanding an immediate search for the cause.

Do you have an itching around your anus (rectal area)?
This is a maddening symptom called pruritis ani, and is caused by foods, medications, vitamins and lotions, but can often result from hemorrhoids, fistula (opening from the interior of the rectum to the skin), fissure (crack in the anal area) and benign and malignant skin conditions. More serious rectal diseases such as cancer must be ruled out. Persistent or recurrent pruritis ani demands a thorough diagnostic evaluation.

Do you experience difficulty in swallowing? There are two types of swallowing difficulty, so a distinction must be made between them. If you have difficulty swallowing liquids and solids alike you may be suffering from an esophageal motility problem, a failure of your esophagus to propel the food down to your stomach. On the other hand, if you have had difficulty swallowing solids, which gradually worsens and then involves difficulty swallowing liquids as well, you may have a mechanical obstruction, usually caused by a stricture (narrowed esophagus from scarring due to gastroesophageal reflux), or esophageal cancer. There are many neurological disorders that may cause dysphagia due to esophageal motility disorders and there are also other causes of mechanical obstruction. Dysphagia is a symptom that also demands immediate investigative evaluation.

CLINICAL EXAMPLES

A sixty year old anesthesiologist and his wife went on vacation to the South Pacific islands. They relaxed on the beach, communed with the natives and happily enjoyed the exotic foods. Shortly after they returned home they developed diarrhea, flatulence and cramping abdominal pain. They attributed the symptoms to "changing diets," and decided to wait a while until their "intestinal tract readjusted." But it didn't. When seen in the office, their only physical finding was some upper abdominal tenderness. Stool cultures were ordered and an intestinal protozoa (Entamoeba histolytic), which causes amebiasis (infection with amoeba) was found. Proper therapy resolved their problem quickly.

Twenty years ago, a fifty-five year old woman and her husband were involved in an automobile accident. They were brought to the emergency room of a hospital and evaluated. The woman complained of back pain. X-rays were taken and were normal. She was sent home and her back pain slowly improved. Approximately one week later she suddenly collapsed. She was rushed to the hospital and was found to have a ruptured spleen. Ruptured apparently during the accident, but missed at the time of initial examination. The spleen must have bled slowly over time until it finally clinically reached a very dangerous point. Emergency surgery was performed, the spleen was removed and she received multiple blood transfusions. She made an uneventful recovery. Many months later she was seen in my office for the first time. Her current chief complaint was "weakness and loss of appetite." She told me about her accident and surgery and blood transfusions. This brought to mind the possibility of chronic hepatitis as a result of the blood transfusions. The physical examination was unremarkable, but the blood tests showed some abnormal liver enzymes. She was evaluated for hepatitis and proved to have hepatitis C. On occasion hepatitis C can resolve, but of all the varieties of hepatitis, hepatitis C has the highest rate of chronicity (75%). It can eventually lead to liver failure and liver cancer, but twenty years later—the patient is fine.

Genitourinary

Do you have pain on urination? Do you experience a burning sensation when you urinate? Do you have the urge to go frequently? A yes answer to any of these questions could mean that you have a urinary tract infection.

Have you noted a red or tea colored urine? If so you could be bleeding, and the cause could be a urinary stone, an infection (bacterial, fungal, or tuberculosis), trauma or a benign or malignant tumor someplace in your urinary tract.

Has your urine changed color? Again blood could be the cause, or the color change (dark like tea) could also be a sign of jaundice.

Have you experienced incontinence—that is sudden, unexpected loss of urine? Infection or neurological disorders may be the cause.

Do you awaken at night to urinate? Nocturia could be due to benign or malignant prostate enlargement, urinary bladder problems, cardiovascular disorders, or diuretic medication.

Have you experienced difficulty starting your urinary stream? Do you have to strain or exert lower abdominal pressure to start the stream? Has your urinary stream narrowed or become weaker? Do you experience dribbling? If the answer to any of these questions is yes, you may be experiencing prostatic enlargement or urethral stricture (blockage).

CLINICAL EXAMPLES

When I was a resident at Cook County Hospital (making 125 dollars a month) the evenings I wasn't on call, I did some moon-lighting at a local clinic. The neighborhood I worked in was an economically deprived part of the city. On one occasion, an eighteen year old came to the clinic complaining of a "yellowish urethral discharge." Yes, those were his exact words when I elicited his chief complaint. This was enough for me to pay strict attention, because the descriptions I would usually get for this particular chief complaint were words not found in Webster's dictionary. Yes, he had made his own diagnosis, describing it as gonorrhea as opposed to the "clap" of his peers. My lecture on safe sex was met with a knowing nod of his head, and a discourse that stunned me because of his vocabulary, which I would have expected to hear on the Harvard University campus. He received his penicillin and was presumably cured. So I was surprised when he showed up again a month later—yes, you guessed it—with the same diagnosis. This time we extended our conversation, and I suggested to him that he needed to make some better choices. He agreed, fully admitting that the ladies with whom he was associating were prone to such diagnosis as opposed to what he might run into if he selected, for instance, some high society debutantes. I also extended the conversation to suggest that he was of an intellectual bent, and seemed to be intelligent enough that when he completed High School, I hoped he would attend college. "You can be sure of that," he said. Now I know you probably will not believe me when I tell you I saw him once again—yes, you guessed it—with the same diagnosis. We spoke more, by this time adding to the rapport that we had developed. Skip now six years ahead. I was well established in practice, and into my office strolls this gentleman, well dressed in a suit and silk tie, cashmere (I think) overcoat, immaculate, shoes polished like the military. Yes, it was my old friend. "Just thought I'd say hello, doc." We spoke for a while and he took me outside to see his brand new Cadillac parked in the parking lot. "I did what you told me, doc." Smiling proudly, I said, "I'm really glad you came to see me. I'm proud of you. Thanks for coming." He nodded and said, "Uhh—I got a problem, doc." Yes, you guessed it!

A middle aged healthy man injured his shoulder. He was experiencing considerable pain. His wife has severe rheumatoid arthritis and was taking a non-steroidal anti inflammatory medicine. I forget the exact name of the powerful one she was taking, but you are familiar with the milder ones in this family—motrin or advil. He came to the hospital emergency room. His chief complaint was weakness, loss of appetite, nausea and vomiting. He felt he was "dehydrated" and it dawned upon him that he had not passed any urine for "a while." When I asked if he was on any medicines, he said no, but his wife pointed out that he had taken "one of my rheumatoid arthritis pills for his shoulder." This still didn't register much with me, but stat blood studies revealed evidence of uremia—kidney failure otherwise known as renal failure. Then the significance of his uremia became evident. He had developed acute renal failure from taking *one* of his wife's pills. What happened to this gentleman was a rare, but known, complication of the non-steroidal class of drugs—kidney shutdown. He had to undergo acute renal dialysis treatments, and made a full recovery.

Gynecological

Menstrual history should include questions about the age of onset of your menstrual periods, the frequency of periods, the duration of your period, the number of pads used per day, pain during your periods, occurrence of menopause. These questions are geared to determine normalcy, or whether there is a menstrual or post-menopausal problem, the causes of which could be gynecological or related to other medical problems.

Do you have a vaginal discharge? Discharges are more often than not due to an infection, (bacterial or yeast) but could be caused by a malignancy.

CLINICAL EXAMPLES

A twenty some year old Mexican lady was brought to the hospital as an emergency with severe vaginal bleeding. She spoke very little English, but did manage a chief complaint of "My boyfren gooz me wid fonnypaper." "What did you say?" a friend of mine, and fellow intern, asked. She repeated herself again. Not understanding what she meant, he placed her on the examining table and examined her. The diagnosis was made immediately. Her chief complaint was accurate. In an attempt to abort his girlfriend's early pregnancy, her boyfriend had rolled up the Chicago Tribune's comic pages into a firm rod and inserted it into her vagina thinking he could end the pregnancy. All he accomplished was a severe vaginal laceration, which my friend successfully sutured. This was in the days before Roe V. Wade when amazingly novel and often dangerous methods were invented for the purpose of inducing abortion, including the use of potassium permanganate. This method was by far the most common, and the most dangerous. It was either self induced or friend assisted. This toxic chemical was often incorrectly used, as I found out when a patient was brought to the emergency room in shock. She had placed potassium permanganate directly in her vagina and succeeded in destroying her pelvis including her bladder, and some intra abdominal intestinal contents. She did not survive emergency surgery.

During my internship at Cook County Hospital, I delivered a twenty-two year old of a healthy seven pound girl—her eleventh child. She informed me that with all her pregnancies and breast feedings she had never had a menstrual period—she did, however, clearly understand the reasons why.

Endocrine

The endocrine system includes the major glands of the body. These glands secrete more than twenty hormones into the blood stream that regulate many bodily functions. Hormones are chemicals that are carried by the blood stream to different cells of the body and act upon them. The endocrine glands include the hypothalamus of the brain (that part of the brain that includes vital autonomic regulatory centers and is connected to and controls the pituitary gland), thyroid gland, parathyroid glands (four—imbedded in the thyroid), adrenal glands, pineal body, pituitary gland and ovaries and testes. In addition, the stomach, intestines, liver, heart and pancreas, in part, also serve an endocrine function by secreting hormones into the blood stream.

Dysfunction of any endocrine gland can result in a multiplicity of symptoms, too numerous to do justice in a short review. In general, the changes that occur in the body as a result of over or under functioning of an endocrine gland may be subtle and difficult to diagnose in the early stages. Questions related to history of growth, weight changes, constipation, changes in hand and foot size, head size, changes in your pulse rate, skin pigmentation, energy levels, skin dryness, intolerance of heat or cold, sterility, thirst, increased urination, impotence and tremor can provide clues to an endocrine disorder.

Your physician can be alerted to the possibility of diabetes if you complain of thirst and increased urination. These are late symptoms. Are you intolerant to heat and cold? If so this may indicate thyroid disease.

CLINICAL EXAMPLES

A patient asked me if I would see his mother. She was an eighty-six year old resident of a nursing home, and he said he "was watching her die slowly, and I want to be sure that everything is being done for her." He was willing to bring her to my office in a wheel chair. She was sent to the nursing home with the diagnosis of Alzheimer's disease. I told him I would be happy to see her, but I didn't want to build up false hopes because there was very little to offer Alzheimer's patients in those days. He understood, thanked me and brought her to the office. She was a tiny lady with thin, and sparse white hair and what I'm sure would have been beautiful, sparkling blue eyes many years ago. She sat in the wheel chair with head and upper body stooped over. When I said hello to her, she very slowly lifted up her head (it was like watching a movie run in slow motion), looked at me, and spoke. Her word or words were unintelligible. Her voice was very hoarse and she sounded like a creaking frog. With the slow motion and the attempt at speech the diagnosis was made. Her skin was dry and flaking, and her reflexes demonstrated a phenomenon known as delayed relaxation phase. When you strike with a reflex hammer—take the biceps reflex for example—the arm should jerk up and down equally and rapidly (more later under physical examination—neurology). In the patient's case the arm jumped up quickly, but the down phase was very slow, described as delayed relaxation phase of the deep tendon reflex. All these physical findings were characteristic of hypothyroidism in the extreme, known as Myxedema, and unless treated would lead to coma and death. She was started on thyroid replacement therapy—extremely tiny doses at first with slight increases every three weeks. To make a long story short, she slowly improved, regained some strength and mental capability. She lived for four more years and was able to communicate much better with her family.

A thirty-six year old woman developed hypertension in her last month of pregnancy. She delivered a healthy girl, but her high blood pressure did not resolve, so she embarked upon a long quest to get her blood pressure under control. She experienced intermittent success, but more often than not, her blood pressure remained elevated in spite of the wide variety of medications that were tried, and in spite of embarking upon a vigorous exercise program, including many ten and fifteen kilometer races coupled with a thirty seven pound weight loss. The patient also had a serum potassium level lower than normal. The combination of resistant hypertension and low blood potassium should have alerted her doctors to a major problem, but they attributed this combination more to a side effect of the medicines than anything else. The patient did her own Google searches and learned that when a blood pressure could not be brought under control, in spite of intensive therapy, a search for a specific and unusual cause should be undertaken. Most (over 90%) of blood pressure patients can be easily controlled with life style changes and/or medications taken by a cooperative patient. Google went on to tell her that a blood pressure elevation with a low potassium demands a careful search for two different types of adrenal gland tumors. She convinced her doctors to order the tests. They did, and unfortunately unequivocal test results gave the patient no satisfaction because the lab personnel had found an unlabelled twenty-four hour urine sample and "assumed it was hers." Needless to say, this made her angry and over the next year the tests were repeated, but the results were still "not enough for anyone to make a firm diagnosis." She even saw an endocrinologist who told her she did not have an adrenal gland problem. The patient persisted, however, and finally, after begging for a referral from her HMO doctor, was sent to a cardiologist who finally ordered a CT scan of the adrenal glands, and there they were, not one—but two adrenal tumors! This started her on a search for the appropriate therapy, including seeing a world authority from the University of Oklahoma, and I won't go into the incredible details of all the surgical options open to her, but there was one medical option available, that after much soul-searching and personal research she chose—and that was to take a forty year old medicine that would effectively block the excess hormone that her adrenal tumors were pouring out and that caused the potassium loss and hypertension. Taking the medication faithfully has resulted in a normal blood pressure and a normal serum potassium. This is a perfect example of a patient taking charge of her healthcare!

Hematologic

Have you ever had anemia? Were you told that your blood count was low? If so, what was the cause? Was it treated? Have you ever had any blood problems such as Leukemia? Do you bruise easily? Have you ever had abnormal bleeding? Have you had abnormal swelling of your lymph glands? A yes response to any of these questions will alert your physician to many diagnostic possibilities that will require specific studies.

CLINICAL EXAMPLES

A fifty year old woman came to my office for the first time. She had recently moved to the area where I practiced. Her chief complaint was leukemia. "Who's been taking care of you," I asked. "The doctors at Northwestern University," she answered. "Are you on therapy now?" I asked. "No, I'm fine." "Are you in remission?" "If that's what you want to call it, but I've been okay for seven years." I gave her a complete examination and there were no abnormal findings. "I used to have an enlarged spleen," she said. "Oh," I said, "I would like to get some blood tests and a blood count, and we'll have you sign for us to get a copy of your records from Northwestern." She agreed. The patient's blood count and all her blood tests were normal. There was no sign of leukemia. The record from Northwestern arrived and proved that she was indeed treated for leukemia. The bone marrow study at the time was confirmatory. In fact she had the type of leukemia that offered a very poor prognosis, but here she was—ten years after diagnosis, and perfectly well. How does one explain this?

A seventy year old lady was seen by me at Cook County Hospital's hematology clinic. Her chart was on my desk and was at least four inches thick. "Wow," I said, "you sure have a thick chart." She told me that she had been coming to Cook County for twenty years. "What for?" I asked. "I got cancer of the liver." Since it wasn't likely that anyone with cancer of the liver would live twenty years in those days, I was incredulous to say the least. So I opened up her chart from the beginning—and there it was. In fact, there were sketches of her liver based on the physical examination findings. They were signed by physicians who had preceded me in the clinic for the last twenty years. Some of these doctors were now my mentors. These drawings showed the edge of an easily palpable, extremely large and knobby liver extending far below her rib cage. Normally the liver is, at best, barely palpable at about the level of the bottom of the rib cage and is very smooth with a clearly defined sharp edge. A liver filled with large nodules is more than likely a cancerous liver. I'm not sure of the date I saw this patient, but since I was at Cook County in the late fifties and early sixties she had to have been diagnosed with cancer in the forties. She did not have the benefit of effective chemotherapy in those days. So what do we have? Could this also be another rare case of spontaneous remission of cancer? When I was in medical school, Dr. Warren Cole, professor of surgery, collected 100 case reports of spontaneous remission of cancer. He wrote a book on the subject, hoping to see if there was some common thread to these cases. There wasn't, so what do we have? Is it divine intervention? Is it a rejuvenated immune system? Is it both? What is it?

Allergic/Immunologic

Have you had recurrent skin rashes, hives, eczema, hayfever, chronic runny nose, redness of the eyes? Do any of these symptoms occur only at certain times of the year? This would suggest a seasonal incidence characteristic of many allergies. Are you known to be sensitive to pollens, mold, dust, danders, certain foods? Although in theory any food can cause a food allergy, the "big eight" foods are incriminated in 90% of cases. These are: milk, eggs, soya, wheat, fish, shellfish (including mussels, crab and shrimp), peanuts from the ground and peanuts from trees (Brazil nuts, hazelnuts, almonds and walnuts).

CLINICAL EXAMPLES

Rather than give a clinical example here, I will discuss some interesting facts about allergies. They are extremely common. In the United States it is estimated that fifteen million people suffer from hay fever, ten million have asthma, and even more are allergic to medications, food and insects. Allergies have a hereditary component. An allergy occurs when your immune system overreacts to a substance (usually harmless) known as an allergen. This allergen enters your body by a number of routes including: skin, nose, lung and digestive tract. Examples of an allergen are: dust, mold, pollen, dander, mites, feathers, foods, drugs and insect stings. This reaction between an allergen and the immune system causes the allergic symptoms. Allergic diseases include: asthma, hayfever, hives, skin rashes and insect stings. The symptoms of these illnesses vary from mild to life threatening. The worst allergic manifestation is known as anaphylaxis and its symptoms include sudden onset of hives, which may include swelling of the throat, breathing difficulty and a sudden drop in blood pressure that could cause death if not promptly treated with epinephrine (adrenalin).

Musculoskeletal

This system includes muscles, ligaments, cartilage, tendons, bones and joints.

Have you had any fractures, dislocations or disabling sprains? Any past bone or joint surgery? Any residual from these injuries? Any joint stiffness or pain? Which joints? Any muscular weakness? Any back pain? You will have no difficulty advising your physician of the specific musculoskeletal problem you are experiencing.

CLINICAL EXAMPLES

A seventy year old man was seen with a chief complaint of urinary difficult. He didn't empty his bladder, he was awakened three or four times per night to urinate and his urinary stream was narrow and slow. As part of his musculoskeletal system review it was also learned that he complained of aching and stiffness of both thighs and hips that was worse in the morning, and improved as the day wore on. Tests were ordered, but he never got them because he developed urinary obstruction and was urgently admitted to the hospital. He was seen in consultation, by a urologist who performed prostate surgery to relieve the blockage. While in the hospital it was noted that he was moderately anemic. This finding, taken together with his morning hip stiffness, raised the possibility of a disorder know as polymyalgia rheumatica. This was confirmed by a blood test known as a sedimentation rate, which was 400% higher than normal. The cause of the disorder is unknown. It responds to therapy with low dose cortisone.

Here is another example of a secondary diagnosis resulting from a carefully taken system review.

A thirty-six year old woman was seen complaining of severe back pain. It had slowly developed and reached the point where the pain became persistent and varied with position. She couldn't lie flat or on her back and right side, and was only able to sleep in a reclining position. A complete physical examination was performed, and the only other finding was a slightly retracted area of the skin of the right breast under which was a deep two centimeter mass, not readily palpable, but visible by mammography ordered because of the skin retraction. The two were connected. The mass was malignant and an X-ray of the spine, ordered because of the pain, showed evidence of widespread metastases.

Neurologic

Questioning in the neurological part of the system review can be divided up into anatomical categories.

Cranial nerves (nerves originating in your brain and extending to the head and neck):

Have you lost your sense of smell, or have you noted any change in your ability to smell? (Cranial nerve 1—olfactory).

Have you noted any visual disturbances (focusing—double vision)? (Cranial nerves 2,3,4,6—optic, occulomotor, trochlear, abducens).

Have you noted any strange sensations around your mouth and difficulty chewing? (Cranial nerve 5—trigeminal).

Have you experienced a change in your ability to taste foods? (Cranial nerve 7—facial).

Are you experiencing any hearing difficulties or disturbances of your equilibrium? (Cranial nerve 8—auditory, also called vestibulocochlear).

Have you noted any speech difficulties, swallowing problems and taste problems? (Cranial nerves 9,10,12—glossopharyngeal, vagus, hypoglossal).

Has there been a change in your ability to move your neck or turn your head? Cranial nerve 11—accessory).

I can't resist giving you a mnemonic here that all medical students have used to remember the cranial nerves, and that has been in use for centuries. (On old Olympus's towering tops a Finn and German viewed some hops.) I'm not sure if the mnemonic has been ruined when the name of the auditory nerve was changed to vestibulocochlear?

Motor system (movement).

Have you ever had paralysis, convulsions, involuntary movements, change in your ability to use your legs, or your arms? Have you noted any lack of coordination in any of your movements?

Sensory system (feeling).

Do you have sudden pains or lightening pains? Have you experienced a total or partial lack of feeling (numbness) of any part of your body? Have you experienced increased sensations or increased sensitivity of any part of your body?

Autonomic nervous system: (that part of the nervous system that controls internal functions of the body and is not under your conscious control).

Have you experienced a change in your ability to differentiate cold from warm? Have you had any change in your ability to sweat? Have you noted any change in the color of your skin—redness or blueness? Have you had any problem with bowel or bladder control?

Positive responses to any of the above questions related to the different parts of your nervous system could lead your physician to a precise localization of brain, spinal cord, peripheral and autonomic nervous system pathology.

CLINICAL EXAMPLES

I received a phone call from a patient who advised me that his unconscious wife was being transported to the hospital, and would I please see her. I didn't know his wife, so I was completely unfamiliar with her medical history. When I saw her, she was immobile, could not move her arms or legs or any other part of her body, but was able to move her eyes. Amazingly enough she had retained cognitive function and was able to blink her eyes in response to questioning. That was the only part of her face and body that could move. I called a neurologist to see the patient who diagnosed a stroke—specifically located in the pons, an area in the brain stem that relays messages between the cerebral cortex, the cerebellum and the spinal cord. This clinical syndrome is also known as the locked-in syndrome, reflecting what is actually happening. The patient is completely immobile (except for her eyes) and is locked in her own paralyzed body. "What's the prognosis?" I asked the neurologist in private. "She'll never recover and most patients do not live more than a month." Then he shook his head and said, "If that ever happens to me, be kind—do away with me." The patient remained in the hospital for about two weeks, and then was transferred to a nursing home for further supportive care. Now, as Paul Harvey says, comes the rest of the story. Miraculously, this patient recovered to the point of regaining upper body and extremity motion and speech. She progressed to a wheel chair and took her place again on the Board of Directors of a major Chicago corporation where she had previously served.

So much for dogmatic medical prognostication.

A forty-eight year old woman complained of "drooping eyelid and double vision." In addition she noted that after walking, her legs would "get weak, but after I stop and rest they get stronger." These symptoms would occur together and sometimes separately. This is a fairly typical collection of symptoms for a specific neurological illness known as Myasthenia Gravis. It is another in the family of autoimmune illnesses, in this case caused by destruction of chemical receptors on nerve junctions resulting in disruption of nerve impulses. A neurologist confirmed the diagnosis and the patient was started on a drug called pyridostigmine, which again, as in most autoimmune diseases, is not curative, but offers partial to good symptomatic relief.

Psychiatric

Mental health problems include changes in behavior, habits and personality. Social withdrawal effecting ones life is frequent during a mental illness. Some of the more common mental health problems include depression, bipolar disorders (manic depression), schizophrenia, anxiety, panic disorder, post traumatic stress disorder, alcohol or drug abuse dependence disorder, agaraphobia, hyperchondriasis, eating disorder, obsessive compulsive disorder, psychosis and dementia.

The cause of mental illness may be due to environmental stresses; it may be genetic in origin; it may represent reaction to trauma; it may be the result of brain chemical imbalances. It is also possible that susceptibility to mental illness may result from a combination of two or more of these factors. It has been estimated that a third of all primary care physician visits may be related to such disorders. The careful physician will not neglect this part of the medical history. The psychiatric system review is usually saved for the last item, unless the patient's chief complaint is in the mental health realm. If not, by the end of the history taking exercise the physician should have a very good idea of your psychiatric make up. There are numerous mental health question sets dealing with the various psychiatric diagnosis as above mentioned, but these are lengthy, some taking as much as a half hour to complete. In the primary care office setting during an initial patient interview, your physician should end up with a good idea about your degree of depression or anxiety, if any, and whether or not you may fall into one of the mental health diagnostic categories mentioned above.

During the course of my working on a computerized self-administered patient history, I was amazed by the number of patients who pressed yes to the question: Have you ever had any serious suicidal thoughts? This is a question rarely asked during the taking of a complete medical history unless the chief complaint is psychiatric.

CLINICAL EXAMPLE

A four month old Polish-Jewish girl named Doris was brought to the United States in February of 1904 by her parents who fled the pogroms in the czarist Russian controlled Pale of Settlement, a geographic region where Jews were forced to live. She grew up in the United States, at first living in Rochester, New York and then Chicago, Illinois. She completed two years of High School with very high grades ("you could take two or four years of High School, and I went in the line where my girlfriends were and it turned out to be the two year line"). After completing the two years she went to work as a legal stenographer. She was so good that the lawyers she worked for said that she knew more than they did. She married a plumber in her early twenties. "I didn't love him, but my father, who knew his father in the old country, liked him and said he was a good man." Family members related that as a young woman, Doris "saw snakes" and 'acted funny.' Doris also mentioned that as a young woman, she believes she saw God, a man in a flowing white gown and a long white beard standing at the edge of her bed. She also experienced bouts of depression. She had a son who died immediately after childbirth, diagnosed as a "blue baby," the name given to cyanotic congenital cardiac defects for which nothing could have been done in those days. Her second son was born and thrived. But by the time he was a toddler Doris's mental state deteriorated, and she was admitted to a mental hospital with 'depression.' She described this experience as "horrible." "They tied me to the bed. I saw a flame leave my body. It was my soul. I have no soul. How can one live without a soul? How do you die if you already lost your soul?" I don't believe a firm diagnosis was made in those days, and Doris eventually went home to her toddler son who had forgotten who she was, and a family, including a mother and father, two sisters and a brother, all of whom did not know how to cope. In addition, apparently Doris now felt in some way contaminated by the experience, and would not touch anybody or anything in the house with bare hands (including her own son). All this apparently for fear of bringing upon them the curse that had inflicted her. Her husband couldn't cope with her illness and left. They were divorced five years later. The relationship between Doris and her family deteriorated, the household became dysfunctional and bitter arguments ensued as the family had great difficulty in understanding Doris' bizarre behavior. Doris' son grew up in this environment, and he too could not understand his mother who refused to ever touch or hug him. If her son tried to hug his mother, she would cry out in anguish and flee. Nevertheless Doris was able to go back to work as a legal stenographer, and boarded in her parent's home with her son. She did well at work, was very popular with the attorneys who vied for her services, and who labeled her "the queen of LaSalle Street." At home, however, conditions remained unchanged. Doris continued to experience intermittent bouts of depression, but never any more hallucinatory symptoms (if that's what they were). One bout of depression, later in life, required electroconvulsive shock treatments. Her parents died, her son left home, and Doris spent her older years living alone in an apartment. She worked until her seventies, all the while her idiosyncracies never changed. She spent the last eight years of her life in a nursing home, visited weekly by a daughter-in-law, every other week by her son and occasionally by her grandchildren and great grandchildren. In her late eighties she began to develop symptoms of dementia, and as these symptoms progressed her idiosyncracies regressed, so that by the time she died at age ninety two she had been able to hold her son's hand and hug him without a single bit of panic or concern.

For many years I took care of a man and wife. On occasion they would bring their teen-aged daughter to see me for self limited minor illnesses such as sore throats or upper respiratory infections. The young lady had no medical problems requiring chronic care. She was tall, attractive, quiet and reserved. When she graduated High School, I was told by her mother that "she's off to college," and at another time, "she's doing well except she's having boy trouble." The last report I received was that she's "living with her boyfriend in California." Years later, I received a call from her mother asking that I see her daughter, because she had broken up with her boyfriend and arrived home very depressed. When she came to the office with her parents, it was clear that her mother had made the right diagnosis. One could have made that diagnosis from her appearance alone. She had a very gloomy affect, a fixed pessimistic, humorless expression, slumped posture, was lethargic and did not make eye contact. Clearly, she was withdrawn and melancholic. Most of my questions were answered by responses such as, "does it matter?" "Who cares?" "What's the difference?" I completed the interview with a feeling of dread, and I asked her if it would be okay to speak with her parents? "Whatever you want" was her reply. I brought her parents into another office and told them that I agreed with them that their daughter was very depressed, so much so that I would want her to either be seen by a psychiatrist immediately, or even better, let me call one of them and make arrangements for her to be hospitalized, because I felt that she was at risk. They informed me that that's what they had wanted for her, but she had refused. She did however agree to see me when that option was offered by her parents. I told them that I would see what I can do, and I went back to speak to the patient. She refused any intervention by a psychiatrist in spite of her not denying that she was depressed. I ended up negotiating back and forth, and the best we could come up with was that I would start her on an antidepressant and the parents (both reliable people) would watch her closely and report her progress or lack of same. I wrote down the name and telephone numbers of two psychiatrists if she changed her mind. One week later I received a call from the mother. Her daughter had checked into a motel and killed herself. That was a shattering experience. Could I have done more? I am haunted to this day.

Although I have given my two examples under the psychiatric history, I must relate one more as an illustration of towering emotional strength that has remained a stirring model for me.

I never saw this elderly lady without a smile on her face. In all the years I took care of her, and in the face of severe symptoms that worsened as she got older, the only answer I ever received when I asked her how she felt was, "Just fine, doctor." Now it was clear that her multiple illnesses made it impossible for her to feel so well, but that's all I ever heard. She would answer yes to specific questioning about pain, weakness, shortness of breath, etcetera, but the bottom line to her was that she was "just fine." This never changed throughout the years that I took care of her, even when she progressed into advanced congestive heart failure and developed severe breathing difficulty that resisted all my efforts and the efforts of a prominent consulting cardiologist who hospitalized her for end-stage aggressive treatment. No one was able to understand what kept her going—but I think I knew the answer. Finally, in what turned out to be her last hospitalization and while lapsing in and out of coma, she opened her eyes, smiled at me, and moved her hand in a feeble wave. I knew what I would hear when I asked it, but I did anyhow. "How are you?" I said. "Just fine, doctor." she whispered. And in that statement was the secret of her living much longer than anyone would have anticipated. She never perceived herself as sick, or if she did she never wanted her family to perceive it. She could only think of herself as well, and she did so until the last minute of her life, which finally gave out at age eighty-four. She was and is a model that I hope I could be able to emulate.

MEDICAL HISTORY SUMMARY

You have just gone through a communication process with your physician. The communication has been both verbal and nonverbal. The nonverbal includes posture, body language, facial expression and eye contact. You each have evaluated each other in these ways. The most important part of your medical examination has been completed. Hopefully you both have taken the time to understand each other and have paved the way to an ongoing, mutually beneficial relationship. The health problem that you bring to the interview has caused you to be dependent on your physician. This makes you vulnerable, so you must feel a sense of trust in your relationship. You have learned if your physician has the ability to listen. This ability is the key to understanding. You have an idea as to whether your physician has shown empathy, without which you will lose confidence in his ability to care for you. The history taking process is not a one way street. The physician is not the only one who asks questions. You must also query your physician when you are not certain what a question means. Your physician has taken on an awesome responsibility and needs all the help he can get. You must cooperate fully in that process. Nothing must be hidden. When it seems as if the interview has come to a close, the wise physician will ask, "Is there anything else you feel we may not have discussed?" "Are there any questions you would like to ask me?" Have I missed anything you want me to look into?" At the end of the interview your physician has a good idea of the areas necessary to explore in order to come to a diagnosis. At this point in time, incubating in his mind is either a definite diagnosis, or a list of possible diagnosis known as a differential diagnosis. Now a complete physical examination must be done, and the physician has learned, based upon your history, what part of the examination will need special emphasis.

Are you ready for the physical examination now? Good. Let's go.

PART II
THE PHYSICAL EXAMINATION

✦

"Observe, record, tabulate, communicate. Use your five senses."

Sir William Osler
(1849–1919)

INTRODUCTION

The examination room should be well lit, private and quiet. You should be seated upon an examination table so the physician has access to both sides of your body, although most of the examination will take place with the physician standing on your right side. Hopefully, by now, after the history has been taken, your level of anxiety has been reduced to the point where you will fully cooperate during the exam. The physician utilizes the sense of sight, hearing, touch and smell when performing a physical examination. (The sense of taste was used by physicians 100 years ago—tasting urine for sugar—in diagnosing diabetes, but lab testing has made that unnecessary—thank goodness). Yes, there are some diagnoses such as diabetic acidosis that can be smelled from across the room.

These senses are brought to bear utilizing four methods:

Inspection (observing with eyes).

Palpation (touching with hands).

Percussion (percussing with fingers and finger tips).

Auscultation (listening with a stethoscope).

In order for your physician to take full advantage of these four methods you must be undressed, and suitably draped with a paper or cloth gown. I am always amazed when observing a Hollywood movie and watching the actors at work examining a fully clothed patient. How can a physician inspect a clothed body? How does one palpate over clothes? How do you percuss through clothes, and how do you listen carefully with a stethoscope rubbing over clothes and distorting body noises? Modesty has a place, but it cannot interfere with a good physical examination.

Now we'll discuss these four methods.

Inspection

Inspection is a careful visual evaluation of your body—first your entire body and then of each body system as your physician goes through the sequence of events necessary for the performance of an adequate examination. If you observe your doctor staring at you or a part of your body, understand that he is observing you for symmetry, as the two sides of your body are virtually symmetrical. You are also being observed for anything that interferes with that symmetry, whether it is a skeletal deformity or an abnormal growth, or any out of place internal body mass or motion. Much can be learned from careful observation.

Palpation

If your physician has noted anything out of place during the inspection process, or even if he has not, he will palpate different areas. He will also palpate over an organ such as liver or spleen or thyroid gland to determine if there are any enlargements. When your physician palpates, he is utilizing a sense of touch to assess organ location and size, temperature, texture, roughness, swellings of any kind, crepitation (feeling of bubbly air under the skin as seen with a ruptured lung or an infection under the skin), spasticity and pain or tenderness. Your physician will use his whole hand in the process as follows:

The back of his hand to determine temperature differences;

Fingertips to determine the presence of small lumps or pulsations and for more discrete touch discrimination;

The fifth finger side of the hand to determine if there is any vibration;

The pads of the fingertips to grasp any deep-seated lump.

Hopefully your physician has warmed his hands prior to this process. For deeper palpation, such as that needed to probe for internal organs, you will need to be positioned properly and urged to relax your muscles to the best of your ability. Taking a deep breath will facilitate this process.

Percussion

When your physician percusses your body he utilizes short, quick strokes of his fingers in order to assess the size or position of organs, or to determine what is underlying a specific location that ordinarily should not be there (fluid in the lungs—for instance). There are two ways to percuss:

In the direct method, the striking fingers directly contact the body.

In the indirect method the striking fingers of one of the physician's hands strikes the top of the ends of the fingers of the other hand resting on your body.

The latter is by far the most common method and the percussion yields a sound and a slight vibration that the experienced physician can evaluate for normalcy. What is the intensity of the sound? Is it loud or soft? Is it a high-pitched or low-pitched sound? How long does the sound linger? Needless to say this takes considerable experience to master. If percussion is performed over the lungs—filled with air—your physician will hear a louder and longer vibrating sound then if the percussion is over a solid organ such as the liver, which will give a shorter and softer sound. With the advent of new imaging studies, the art of percussion has been de-emphasized; I still feel, however, that in experienced hands, it can lead one on the right path to a diagnosis.

Auscultation

Your physician will listen to your body. Most body sounds are soft enough so that they cannot be heard, but with the use of a stethoscope the sounds can be greatly amplified. The sounds most listened for are heart and blood vessel sounds, lung sounds and abdominal sounds.

As regards the format for doing the physical examination of all the organ systems—there is no set way. Each physician is free to perform the examination in the way that he feels is most meaningful. For the purposes of this book I have chosen the head to toe approach. We will start at the top and work our way down—after we determine your vital signs.

VITAL SIGNS

Height
Weight

A rough estimate to evaluate a person's ideal weight and height is:

For women—start at 100 pounds for five feet in height and five pounds for each inch of height over five feet. Thus a five feet and six inch woman should weigh approximately 130 pounds;

For men—start at 106 for five feet and add six pounds for each inch over five feet. Thus a six foot man should weigh approximately 178 pounds. It has recently been shown that even a small amount of overweight has a negative effect on long-term mortality rates. Also being significantly underweight likewise has a similar effect.

Temperature

The normal temperature is from 96.4 Fahrenheit to 99.4. This depends upon the time of day, amount of exercise, food intake, the menstrual cycle and one's age. In the morning 99.4 would be considered a fever. In the evening it may not.

Pulse

Your pulse may be taken at your wrist (radial artery), or neck (carotid artery).

Rate

Consider the resting pulse rate to be normal at sixty to 100 beats per minute. This is variable, however, as a highly conditioned athlete may have a resting pulse as low as forty. I read once where Bjorn Borg (the great tennis champion) had a resting pulse of thirty-eight. Your average physician will, however, probably not see Bjorn in his office, so any resting pulse rate in the forties or lower in an unconditioned person should prompt a careful evaluation.

Rhythm

Is the pulse rate regular or irregular? Is the tempo an even one? Do you have a sinus arrhythmia where your heart rate speeds up with inspiration and slows down with expiration? This irregularity is rhythmic, and is not unusual in children and adolescents, but would be unusual in an older adult and might demand further scrutiny.

Force

Is your pulse beat forceful or weak and thready? Either way it is a reflection of the amount of blood pumped out of the heart during each beat, and could represent loss of blood (weak and thready pulse). A full and bounding pulse may be observed during anxiety or with exercise, and some unusual heart and vascular conditions.

Respiratory rate

A normal respiratory rate in an adult is 10 to 20 breaths per minute. A reduction in rate may be seen in morphine overdose, diabetic coma and increased intracranial pressure, a result of head trauma or a brain tumor. An increase in rate may be seen in cardiac and pulmonary problems, aspirin overdose, or conditions changing the acidity of the blood such as diabetic acidosis. There are also some abnormal respirations such as Cheyne-Stokes respirations where your breaths wax and wane in a regular pattern, decreasing in rate and depth and then increasing. This respiratory pattern occurs with severe heart failure, kidney failure, meningitis, increased intracranial pressure, and can be seen during sleep in the elderly. Another abnormal respiratory pattern is Biot's respirations, which is similar to Cheyne-Stokes except that the pattern is irregular. A series of normal respirations are followed by a period of no breathing that can last as little as ten seconds to as long as a minute. This can occur with heat stroke, head trauma and brain infections. Usually your physician will take your respiratory rate without your knowledge by counting the breaths during a thirty second interval.

Blood Pressure

Blood pressure is the force or pressure of the blood against the blood vessel wall. It consists of two numbers: systolic blood pressure (the pressure of the blood during the contraction phase of the heart—systole), and diastolic blood pressure (the resting pressure that the blood exerts against the blood vessel wall during the resting, or filling phase of the heart beat—diastole). The upper range of normal blood pressure has changed over the last fifty years: from 160 over 90 to 140 over 90 to the current gold standard of 120 over 80. This makes belated sense to me because years back I often wondered why the nonagenarians that I would examine seemed always to have a blood pressure of 110 or less over 70 or less. That's why they became nonagenarians—no doubt.

Your blood pressure is determined by blood output of your heart during each beat (cardiac output), resistance in your blood vessels to the flow of blood (peripheral arterial resistance), total volume of your circulating blood, thickness of your blood (viscosity), and elasticity of the blood vessel walls.

For whatever reason, blood pressure is higher in blacks than whites. It rises as your weight increases. Stress and emotion raises blood pressure. Exercise normally raises blood pressure, which should return to baseline reading within five minutes after the exercise is over. High salt diets may increase blood pressure—as does smoking.

If your blood pressure is abnormally high in the arms, it should also be taken in the thigh to rule out the possibility of a coarctation of the aorta (congenital narrowing of the aorta), which decreases the flow of blood to the legs (this is a rare condition).

If your blood pressure is determined to be elevated, it must be treated by lifestyle changes, weight loss, low salt diet, cessation of tobacco use and exercise. Medication may be necessary and is vital if the blood pressure elevation persists after serious life style changes. Those few patients who fail to respond to the usual drug therapy should be investigated for rare causes of high blood pressure such as two different types of adrenal gland tumors and kidney artery blockage.

CLINICAL EXAMPLES

Many diagnoses are made by simply measuring the vital signs. The patient whose weight is much greater than expected based upon height is suffering from obesity. With all the increased morbidity and mortality from this disease, corrective measures are a must. A patient with an elevated temperature probably has an infection, but also could have many other forms of illness. Any temperature that does not resolve within a week or two must be investigated thoroughly. The patient whose pulse beat is irregular in rate and force probably has atrial fibrillation. If this arrhythmia is proven by an electrocardiogram, therapy must be instituted as soon as possible. There are many other forms of cardiac irregularity that can be diagnosed by examining the pulse. An altered or increased respiratory rate in the absence of a fever demands an explanation.

SKIN, HAIR AND NAILS

Skin

Ordinarily your physician will evaluate your skin as he goes through the various parts of your examination, but for the purpose of clarity I will discuss the skin, hair and nails exam fully in this section. You may have told your physician that there have been no changes to any moles, but now he will carefully recheck your impression. Measurements in millimeters of any lesion may be taken in order to have a baseline for future comparisons.

Your physician will concentrate on the color of your skin as follows:

General pigmentation—increased in Addison's disease (adrenal gland insufficiency);

Areas of vitiligo—complete loss of pigment—an autoimmune disorder where your immune system rejects normal body pigment cells;

Yellow jaundice—a sign of liver, gall bladder, pancreatic disease or a blood disorder known as hemolysis where certain illnesses or medications cause destruction of red blood cells.

Pallor—pale or white skin as a result of severe anemia;

Cyanosis—a bluish mottling of the skin resulting from oxygen poor blood that can be seen with pulmonary diseases, cardiac failure and anemia;

Color changes will be difficult to evaluate in dark skinned individuals.

Your physician will evaluate the degree of hydration of your skin. Very dry, cracked skin could be a sign of dehydration.

Hair

Inspection and palpation of the hair can lead to important clues. Thin, fine hair can be seen in hypothyroidism. Excessive hair growth (head and body) can be seen with adrenal and testicular malignancies and pituitary gland hyperactivity. Absent genital hair suggests an endocrine gland abnormality. Male pattern hair loss is common, and most men experience it to varying degrees during their life time. There are many other causes of hair loss. Some are temporary such as occur

74

some months after a major illness or surgery and is felt to be stress induced. You may lose hair both with an underactive and an overactive thyroid. Certain medications can cause hair loss: chemotherapy agents, birth control pills, antidepressants, anticoagulants and too much vitamin A.

Fungal infection of the scalp can cause localized hair loss. Some chronic illnesses such as diabetes can cause unexpected hair loss. Physicians are seeing more hair loss as a result of tight pigtails, tight hair rollers and cornrows. If these methods cause scarring of the scalp the hair loss could be permanent.

Nails

Careful inspection of the nails is a must. They are a mirror to systemic disease. Specifically, your physician will look for changes of shape or growth and changes in color.

The shape changes or growth changes include:

Clubbing (puffing out of the entire nail)—seen in many chronic lung diseases and including cancer, congenital heart disease and inflammatory bowel disease;

Pitting—seen in psoriasis;

Spooning (concave depression of the nails)—seen in iron deficiency anemia;

Separation of the end of the nail from the nail bed—seen in hyperthyroidism.

Color changes and nail lines are indicative of a long list of unusual diseases, poisonings, infections, autoimmune diseases, malignancies and organ failure.

CLINICAL EXAMPLES

A friend of mine called me on the phone one day when I was making rounds in the hospital. He told me about a good friend of his who was ill and getting worse in spite of medical attention. "He's weak and got a fever that won't quit. They told him he has the flu, but I think it's lasting too long." "Yes, I'd be happy to see him," I said, "bring him to the outpatient department." The gentleman was in his fifties, well dressed with suit and tie and a full head of black hair. The patient's vital signs were normal except for a borderline elevated pulse rate of 100 and a temperature of 100.4. Another positive physical finding was an audible cardiac murmur picked up by stethoscope. This was not enough to make a diagnosis, because one could see many patients who happen to have fever from a flu virus and a long standing murmur that has nothing to do with the flu. But the clincher resided in the patient's fingernails. He had what is known as splinter hemorrhages under his nails (long thin lines of blood). This unusual finding is diagnostic for subacute bacterial endocarditis, a serious bacterial infection of a heart valve, uniformly fatal if left untreated. The combination of the murmur, fever and splinter hemorrhages raised a strong index of suspicion. His blood culture was positive for bacteria, and this was enough to prove the diagnosis. I called up a doctor who I knew at the hospital the patient lived near and arrangements were made to hospitalize him. He responded to massive doses of penicillin for six weeks. When he was felt to be bacteria free, he underwent open heart surgery and made an uneventful recovery. Interestingly enough, even though he was treated with the penicillin and his blood cultures were free of bacteria, when his damaged heart valve was taken out and replaced with a new valve, the old valve still grew out some of the organisms. This shows how resistant to medical therapy some of these infections can be. It was knocked down, but not out. The patient made a full recovery and did well.

A twenty-seven year old man came to the office with the chief complaint of a "changing mole." The mole was located on the lateral right shoulder area overlying the upper deltoid muscle. It measured 1⅛ centimeters, was very dark brown to black (he hadn't noticed the blackness before), had irregular borders and had elevated "higher than it was." He had the mole since he was a teenager, but recently noticed the change and was aware of the "warning signs." The lesion was consistent with a melanoma, and he was referred to a surgeon. A wide incision was made, the lesion was removed, and the diagnosis was confirmed. Happily, this young man, the son of a friend, is now forty-two years old and is well. He gets yearly skin examinations from the surgeon, and avoids the sun or uses sunscreen if he can't.

HEAD

Your physician will use inspection and gentle palpation of your head in an attempt to find any scalp lumps (tumors or cysts) or tender spots that could be indicative of infection. If anything is found by palpation, your physician will have to visually inspect so as to diagnose the lesion. On rare occasions auscultation of the head may uncover various types of blood vessel malformations when a faint bruit (blood vessel noise) is heard.

CLINICAL EXAMPLES

An examination of the scalp in a sixty seven year old man demonstrated a one centimeter firm mass about two inches above the right ear. It was not freely movable and was non tender. The mass was removed and it revealed a malignancy—clearly metastatic from a distant site. A chest X-ray showed the primary site of origin to be the lung.

An eighty year old man developed hematuria (blood in the urine). This demands a urological investigation and the urologist cystoscoped the patient (looked into his urinary bladder). He found cancer. The patient underwent surgery and chemotherapy. He saw me on a follow up visit, complaining of lumps on his skin and head. The lumps were small, pea to bean sized, and proved to be metastatic from his bladder cancer. He had made his own diagnosis, calmly saying, "I think the cancer sent out some seeds."

EYES

Your physician can perform a screening examination of your eyes. The principle tools necessary are your physician's own eyes—to inspect external anatomy, and an ophthalmoscope to inspect internal anatomy. By observing your eyes it is possible to determine if you have visible redness and discharge indicating an infection of your conjunctiva (transparent protective covering of the exposed part of your eyes). Shining a light in your eye will tell your physician if your pupils react equally and quickly. This is a reflex beyond your conscious control. Failure to react reflects a neurological problem that will require investigation. The shining light may also demonstrate whether you have cataracts (a cloudiness of your lenses interfering with vision). A slight difference in pupil size (anisocoria) in the absence of any other findings is not uncommon and considered normal. By pulling down your lower eyelids a rough determination can be made as to whether you are anemic. Normally the lower conjunctiva should be red, reflecting the amount of blood brought to the area. A pale conjunctiva could mean you are anemic. There are six muscles which attach the eyeball to its orbit. They allow the eyeball to move in different directions, and are under the control of three cranial nerves. By telling you to "hold your head steady and follow my fingers," your physician can determine if your intraocular muscles are working normally. Again, if they are not, a neurological disorder is present. Other examinations your physician may be able to do are:

A test for color-blindness using the familiar Ishihara color-blind test book;

A test of visual acuity using the familiar Snellen eye chart;

A visual fields test measuring the extent of one's peripheral vision, which if impaired could be indicative of a pituitary tumor or other central nervous system pathology.

An ophthalmoscope is a vital tool for your physician. It allows him to look inside your eyes. Assuming you have no cataracts that are opaque to light, by looking into your eyes your physician can visualize your retina (the visual receptive layer of the eye where light waves are changed into nerve impulses that travel through the optic nerve to the brain—and give you sight). One of the retinal structures is the optic disc (the start of the optic nerve). This structure normally appears white and circular with clearly defined borders (there are some anatomical variations that are considered normal). If the borders are not clearly defined, but rather are hazy, it may be a sign of increased intracranial pressure as seen with a brain tumor. But by far the most important information that can be gleaned from the ophthalmoscopic exam is the observation of the veins and arteries that lie on the retina. This is the only place where arteries and veins can actually be visualized. Use of the ophthalmoscope makes it possible to diagnose hardening of the arteries, diabetes, optic nerve atrophy (partial or complete death of the optic nerve), high blood pressure, arteriosclerosis, subacute bacterial endocarditis, macular degeneration (the cause of progressive blindness in the elderly), and other local and systemic diseases.

CLINICAL EXAMPLES

I worked at Cook County Hospital as an attending physician on one of the male medicine wards. The responsibility of an attending physician was to see problem patients with the residents and interns and offer advice. I arrived on the floor and was taken to see a patient who had an enlarged liver and spleen and whose diagnosis was obscure. He had just been admitted and was undergoing a diagnostic workup. On the way to see him, we walked by an elderly man sitting in a wheelchair. The patient had a shaggy white beard and disheveled grey hair—what there was of it. He was wearing a white gown opened in the back and was staring straight ahead obviously unaware of his surroundings. He had such a doleful expression that I could not help but stop and ask the group about the elderly gentleman. "Oh, he's just waiting for nursing home placement," said one of the residents. "What's wrong with him?" I asked. "He's senile." I inquired, "Who saw him first? Did anyone get a history?" "I saw him," said the intern. "No one was with him. He was found wandering the street, and was brought here by the police. He couldn't answer any questions. He was confused, so we weren't able to get a history. That's all we know," It became apparent to me that a diagnosis had been made on this elderly man without the rudiments of a good physical examination, for there was a clinical finding that anyone could observe, and apparently had been missed or ignored. (I hoped not the latter). This is one of the dangers in a large city hospital where patients are admitted through the emergency room at a rapid rate, and sometimes overwhelm the medical profession by sheer force of numbers. I can remember the times when I was an intern and would admit and work-up a dozen patients a shift. This patient had one pupil much larger than the other. Now, a slight difference in pupil size can be a normal variant—but not this amount of size difference. This finding is an important neurological sign, especially when the enlarged pupil did not react to light. I asked that they all take a close look. When they did, I also suggested an immediate neurosurgical consultation, because clearly this patient must have sustained a head injury and was suffering from a subdural hematoma, which is an accumulation of blood under the dura mater (the outer lining over the brain). As the blood continues to leak, the hematoma enlarges, presses on the brain and could cause death if not surgically removed. To make a long story short, the diagnosis was confirmed, surgery was performed and the patient markedly improved. The residents and interns learned a lesson. They received no criticism from me. No one will ever be mistake free in this profession. The lesson was enough. It is unlikely that they will ignore pupil size in a confused man again.

And another aspect to that lesson is that doctors are all human, and like other humans *can* make bad judgements—and that is why every patient (if they are able) must be actively involved in directing their healthcare.

I saw a thirty-eight year old man for the first time when he came to my office for a pre-employment physical examination. He was in excellent health and passed the physical, except for one finding that I could not explain. I held up my ophthalmoscope and said, "Has anyone ever looked into your eyes like I did with this instrument?" He shook his head and said, "I don't remember anyone doing that?" "Is your vision okay? I asked. "I have no problem," he answered. "Did you ever wear glasses?" I asked. "No, did you see something wrong in there?" "Yes, I did," I told him, "but frankly I don't know what it is I'm looking at. Let me run a quick check of your vision." I took him into another room, and he passed the Snellen chart easily—20/20 in both eyes. "No problem," I said." "Whatever you have there hasn't interfered with your vision and won't interfere with your work, but since I've never seen it before I would like you to see an eye doctor, just to be sure it's nothing significant." He agreed. What I saw was two irregularly rounded, small, pure white spots lying on the peripheral retina. The patient did visit an ophthalmologist, and was told that the diagnosis was histoplasmosis of the eye, or "histo spots." Histoplasmosis is a fungus, known as histoplasma capsulatum, commonly found in the dust and soil, mostly around the Mississippi and Ohio river. Studies have shown that the majority of adults living in the area are carriers. They have inhaled the spores dropped on the dirt by birds and bats. After the spore is inhaled, it can end up anyplace in the body, but the bodies immune system prevents this. However, the spore does have a tendency to end up in the eye where finally, out of the soil and in a friendly nutritionally adequate environment, it activates and causes disease. If the patient is unlucky the spore will end up in the central retina where it could activate and cause a blind spot. On inhalation of the spores, some do get a mild flu like illness that is transient and passed off as "a virus." Those with a compromised immune system could get a full blown systemic case involving multiple organs. I saw a few more histo spots during the rest of my career, but on those occasions I could make my own diagnosis.

This illustrates that physicians never stop learning new things. Also, it illustrates that you may have the bad luck to come up with a problem that your doctor will not recognize. If you have become an educated patient, you can help him.

EARS

Your ear is a sensory organ that causes you to hear and maintain equilibrium. The external ear contains a canal that ends at the eardrum. The eardrum vibrates with the same frequency as the entering sound waves and conducts those sound waves to three ear bones in the middle ear and then to the inner ear and on to the brain. The inner ear contains the internal hearing apparatus and the vestibular (balance) apparatus.

Your physician will use inspection and palpation to examine your ear. The external ear is a not uncommon area for cysts or small cancers of the skin (basal cell or squamous cell carcinomas). If pulling up on your ear causes pain it could indicate an infection of the ear canal. Wax in the ear canal is easily identified. Your physician will use an otoscope that will allow him to peer inside your ear to visualize your canal and eardrum. He will easily be able to identify an infection or perforation of the ear drum.

Screening tests for hearing acuity can be done by use of a tuning fork. Sound waves can be conducted to your brain either by air conduction (the normal route through your ear canal), or bone conduction in which the sound vibrates through your head bones to your brain. If you report diminished hearing in one ear, your physician will make use of the *Weber test*. He will place a vibrating tuning fork in the midline of your skull and ask you if you hear it better in one ear or hear it equally in both ears. The latter is normal. This is a rough test, certainly not as complete as an audiometric evaluation by an audiologist. A second tuning fork test is the *Rinne test*. This test compares bone conduction sound to air conduction. Your physician will first place the vibrating tuning fork on the bone behind your ear. He will then ask you to signal when the sound disappears. At that point he will immediately place the vibrating end of the tuning fork in front of your ear canal. You should still hear the tuning fork. Normally you will hear the sound twice as long by air conduction as you will by bone conduction.

There is one screening test for vestibular (balance) function that your physician can use. It is called the *Romberg test*. You will be asked to close your eyes and stand with both feet together with hands at your side. Your balance should remain steady for twenty seconds. A small amount of swaying is normal. Your physician will stand close to you in the event you lose your balance. This test is also a measure of other central nervous system functions.

CLINICAL EXAMPLES

A sixty-two year old man came to my office with the chief complaint of "I can feel a little lump in my ear. When I put my little finger in my ear to scratch it, I can feel the lump." I confirmed his finding. He had a typically appearing basal cell carcinoma in the ear canal, a rounded lesion with heaped up edges and a central depression. This is a very slow growing malignancy that can be highly destructive locally, but only rarely metastasizes (spreads to a distant site). He underwent Mohs microscopically controlled surgery, where tissue borders are progressively incised until the specimens removed are microscopically determined to be tumor free by a pathologist. The patient is many years past the procedure and has no recurrence in the ear, although follow up examinations have revealed other sites where basal cell carcinomas have formed.

Sometimes patients can take charge of their health to such an extent that they do not need physicians anymore—at least in the early stages of their medical interaction. I received a phone call from a young woman who asked that I refer her to an ear doctor. As an HMO member, she required a referral from her primary care doctor. I asked her why she needed one, and she told me that she was losing her hearing and she was sure she was getting otosclerosis. Now, otosclerosis is a degeneration of the bones in the middle ear to the extent that the bones become spongy and this results in causing one of the bones (stapes) to become fixed. This, in turn, prevents the bone from vibrating, and therefore the sound cannot be transmitted to the brain. Why do you think you've got otosclerosis?" I asked. "My mother has it," she said, "and the same thing is happening to me that happened to her. She had to have surgery." Now that is a precise and to the point medical history and it was good enough for me. I referred her to an ear specialist. The patient called the office of the physician and spoke to his nurse, inquiring as to the physician's experience in performing stapedectomy—a surgical procedure where the non-vibrating stapes bone is replaced with an artificial prosthesis that has an excellent chance of restoring hearing. She learned that the physician did not perform stapedectomy, but his nurse gave her the name of a doctor who does. At this point she was getting frustrated with the system, so she talked to the HMO medical director, explaining to him that she was certain of her diagnosis, she had already saved them money by not coming to my office and not going to the ear doctor's office, and why not just let her go directly to the office of the doctor who performs stapedectomy, since he had the most experience in performing the tests to determine what option was best for the patient: stapedectomy or medical therapy using fluoride and a hearing aid. By this time she knew all there was to know about the disease. Certainly, she knew more than I did. The medical director agreed, and she saw the specialist who did perform a stapedectomy.

She is in the running for the take charge patient of the year award.

NOSE AND SINUSES

Your physician will first check your external nose to search for any lesions or rashes. This area is a not uncommon site for basal or squamous cell skin cancers, especially as it gets direct sun exposure. He will use the same otoscope with a shorter and wider end piece to investigate the interior of your nose. Your central nasal septum should be in the midline between the two nostrils. At times it is deviated to one side or the other and that could cause nasal obstruction. Your nasal mucosa (lining) appears redder than your oral mucosa. This is because more blood vessels are located here so as to warm the air you inhale.

You have three sinuses: frontal, maxillary and sphenoidal. These sinuses are air filled pockets in the facial and head bones that lighten the skull bones, resonate with sound, have the same lining as does the nose and produce mucus that drains into the nasal cavity. Your physician may press above your nose to see if there is any tenderness (suggesting infection) of the frontal sinuses. He may also press under your eyes and adjacent to your nose to see if there is any tenderness overlying the maxillary sinuses. There is also a light that your physician can use in a dark room. Pressing it above your eye and below your eye will illuminate the frontal and maxillary sinuses. Failure of illumination could mean that the sinus is infected. The sphenoid sinus is deep within the skull, behind the nose and not accessible to examination.

CLINICAL EXAMPLES

A man of about thirty-five years of age was seen in my office for an upper respiratory infection. On examination I discovered a large round defect in his nasal septum. It was, I would estimate, about a centimeter in diameter. In zeroing in on this part of his medical history I asked him if he had had nasal surgery. The answer was no. Likewise was the response to questions about trauma, chronic nose picking, cortisone nasal spray use, exposure to toxins, nose ring and a list of rare diseases that might cause a nasal septal defect. This left cocaine use as the remaining etiology that I could think of—to which he confessed.

My wife and I were invited to dinner at our neighbor's house, and there we met a man and wife, friends of theirs that we had not previously met. When the man found out I was a physician, the conversation turned to the state of his medical health—as it so often does. For a year he had experienced nasal symptoms including bloody and purulent nasal discharge. He saw his physician on many occasions and, as he stated, his doctor found that his sinuses were tender and there were "sores" in his nose. Therapy would result in improvement, but the symptoms would recur. On another occasion he was treated for an ear infection, and also a bout of coughing that his physician attributed to a mild pneumonia. To make a long story short, nothing that the doctor could do would result in a permanent cure. His nasal symptoms worsened. Finally he went to see an ear nose and throat physician, whose nurse took the history. "Do you see many patients like me?" my new friend asked the nurse. "No, not many, but enough so that I'm quite sure I know what's wrong." The patient's eyes lit up. "What is it?" he asked. "I'll let the doctor see you," she wisely answered. "He should be here in just a few minutes." This patient had developed an unusual condition known as Wegener's granulomatosis. This is an autoimmune disease that causes inflammation of the upper, and, sometimes lower, respiratory tract. It is an inflammation of blood vessels, which starts in the nasal area and may spread to the lungs and kidneys. The prognosis for this disease has dramatically improved with the use of immunosuppressive agents and cortisone. We saw this gentleman again five years later at the fiftieth wedding anniversary party of our neighbors who had moved out of state. He was free of disease and feeling well.

MOUTH AND THROAT

Your physician will inspect the inside of your mouth and throat using a light source and tongue blade. He will inspect your teeth and gums for any evidence of infection (gingivitis) that could have a significant bearing on your general state of health. The inside of your mouth and throat will be inspected for any lesions on the mucosa, hard or soft palate and jaws. Your tongue will be inspected on its upper and undersurface. Your physician may elect to palpate any lesions detected to determine its consistency or hardness. Is it freely movable or is it immobile?

Three pairs of salivary glands empty into your mouth:

Parotid—in front of your ears;

Submandibular—under your jaws at the angle;

Sublingual—under your tongue.

These glands secrete saliva through ducts that empty into your mouth. Saliva's purpose is three fold: It lubricates food, cleans the mouth mucosa and starts the process of digestion.

Your physician will palpate these glands as they not uncommonly form cysts or tumors or develop stones within their ducts. If any of these glands are tender it could be caused by bacterial or viral infection or duct blockage.

Your throat or pharynx is separated from your mouth by a fold of tissue known as the anterior tonsillar pillar, behind which rests the tonsils—a collection of lymphatic tissue. The back of the throat and tonsillar area is carefully inspected by direct illuminated observation.

While examining in this region, your physician will palpate for thyroid enlargement. The thyroid gland is located in the front of your neck below your Adam's Apple. Ordinarily the gland is not palpable. If it is palpable it indicates that it is enlarged. If tender, it may be an inflamed gland. If enlarged, rocky hard, or lumpy, it may be malignant. In any case, a symmetrically enlarged gland may indicate an overactive thyroid, while other types of enlargements may be accompanied by underactivity.

weeks. There were no other lymph glands palpable, and scalp, ear, nose, throat and mouth examination were normal. I told him that if it doesn't show a decrease in size soon it should be removed. His sister, a nurse, took him to see a surgeon who excised the node. There was no malignancy. The pathologist felt that it was a reactive benign node perhaps from some recent local infection.

CARDIOVASCULAR

This section of the physical examination includes the heart and major blood vessels (arteries and veins). We will take the arteries first. Your physician will use palpation and auscultation to assess the major arteries. He will palpate the arteries in your neck, wrist, feet and possibly the arteries behind your knees and in front of your elbows. The act of palpation will allow your physician to compare the strength of the arterial pulse on both sides of your body (a rough assessment of whether your blood flow is adequate and equal). The pulsation of the arteries should be equal in force. Any deviation could suggest a blocked or partially blocked artery. In addition, the abdominal aorta—delivering blood to your legs and lower part of your body—can also be palpated through your abdominal wall to determine if its beat is forceful. A wider area of pulsation, as felt by your physician's palpating fingers, suggests that an aortic aneurysm (weakening and ballooning out of the artery) is present. Surgery may be required if the aneurysm is large enough.

An abnormal sound (bruit), due to turbulent blood flow, can be heard over an artery with an arterial block. A bruit is a sure sign of a blockage and may demand more definitive tests to evaluate the extent of the block. These harsh noises can be heard in the neck arteries, the abdominal aorta, and possibly even the kidney and brain arteries—or any artery where an aneurysm or significant block has developed.

There are two locations where your physician can evaluate veins, and thereby learn a great deal about your cardiac status. He will inspect the veins in your neck (jugular) while you are lying down at a thirty to forty-five degree angle. These veins are evaluated because they are connected to the right atrium of your heart (the chamber that receives oxygen-depleted blood from your body). If these veins stay dilated and rise as you recline or stand, it is a good indicator of an increase in the pressure and volume of your blood that is entering the right side of your heart—thus indicating right sided heart failure. A second test to identify right heart failure is known as the hepatojugular reflex. By placing his hand over your liver under your right rib cage and pressing for thirty seconds, blood will empty out of the liver into your veins. If the right side of your heart is able to pump this additional blood volume out without difficulty it will show as a transient rise in the jugular vein, which then falls back to normal. If the jugular vein stays elevated the entire time he is pressing, it could mean right heart failure. A second location to evaluate veins is on the back of your hand. When you hold your hand palm down at waist level, normally you will see distended blood filled veins on the back of your hand. As your hand is raised above the level of your heart, with the assistance of gravity, your veins should collapse quickly. If they do not, this is another indicator of right ventricular heart failure. Left ventricular heart failure manifests itself by back pressure to the lungs causing shortness of breath.

The heart exam:

Inspection: Your physician will visually inspect your chest. Signs of cardiac enlargement may be observed by noting your chest heaving at specific locations. Depending upon the site where heaving occurs, it could indicate either right heart enlargement or left heart enlargement (hypertrophy).

Palpation: If you have a thin chest wall your physician will easily be able to palpate the above mentioned heaves. Also, by carefully palpating your anterior chest wall with the palm of his hand, he may feel a vibration (known as a thrill) secondary to a cardiac murmur (more to follow).

Percussion: One can outline heart borders by percussing the chest, but the x-ray is a much more sensitive test, so percussion of the heart has become a lost art. If your physician percusses the front of your chest he is attempting to get a rough estimate of your heart size. An experienced physician can accurately mark out your heart borders by careful percussion.

Auscultation: This is the principal tool used by your physician to evaluate your heart. By listening carefully with a stethoscope he will note your rate and rhythm. Don't be alarmed if he listens long and carefully, for it takes a while to evaluate what your heart is saying. The first heart sound (S1)—the lub in lub-dup—is caused by the closure of the valves between the ventricles and the atria. This sound means that the pumping action of the heart has just started (systole). The second heart sound (S2)—dup in lub-dup—is caused by the closure of the valves between the ventricles and the pulmonary and aortic arteries (diastole). This is the start of the blood entering and filling both ventricles of your heart. There are variations of these sounds and a third (S3) and fourth heart sound (S4), or extra clicks and noises may be heard. These extra sounds may have pathological significance. A gallop rhythm of the heart is when a third or fourth heart sound is audible by stethoscope, so that what you hear is not a lub-dup, but a lub-dup-dup. A louder gallop rhythm is called a summation gallop and combines the third and fourth heart sounds into one louder sound lub-dup-DUP. This occurs with faster heart beats. A gallop rhythm is usually indicative of heart disease. The most common causes are high blood pressure, aortic valve thickening, ventricular scaring or enlargement. They are not always easy to hear. A physician must be sure there is no wax in his ears, and his stethoscope ear pieces are not blocked. The presence of a gallop requires further investigation.

If you have an abnormality (thickening or loosening) of one or more of your heart valves, it may create a blood flow turbulence that causes an abnormal sound called a murmur. Your physician will carefully auscultate to grade and time these murmurs. They are graded by the type and loudness of the sound (grade one through four—faint to very loud). Do these murmurs occur during systole (after the first heart sound), or do they occur in diastole (after the second heart sound)? The murmur, and the location where it is heard best on the anterior chest wall, can lead to a definite diagnosis as regards the heart valve(s) involved. The difficulty here is that not all murmurs indicate heart disease, so it takes an experienced physician to sort this out.

If your physician has not heard, seen, or felt abnormalities, he is in a position to say to you, "I found no abnormalities in your heart exam." This is reassuring to a certain extent, and it means he heard no abnormal heart sounds: S1 and S2 were normal, there was no S3 or S4, or abnormal clicks or murmurs; your heart rate and rhythm were normal; there were no extra beats. Your physician cannot know the extent—if any—of coronary artery narrowing that has not yet given you any symptoms, and this could be true even if your electrocardiogram is perfectly normal. A carefully done heart examination, plus knowledge about your symptoms, your family history, your propensity to cardiac risk factors, can tell your physician if further evaluation is necessary—even if your heart physical exam is normal.

CLINICAL EXAMPLES

When I was a teenager my grandfather was diagnosed with 'heart block.' Your heart is an amazing electrical machine, and each heart beat of the ventricles is started by an electrical impulse that originates in one of the upper heart chambers (atria), prompts the atria to beat, then travels downwards and prompts the lower heart chambers (ventricles) to beat, pumping blood to your body. If this electrical pathway is disrupted completely (usually by scars from a heart attack), the ventricles do not receive their electrical message. The logical question is to ask—then how do they beat? Yes, they do beat by virtue of an intrinsic rhythm of the ventricles that God, in his wisdom built in as a safety valve. This intrinsic rhythm, however, beats at a slower rate, and the rate can get slow enough to cause syncope (fainting spells). In this day and age, a patient exhibiting these symptoms would be fitted with a cardiac electronic pacemaker that will trigger a normal heart rate if it senses a heart rate below a preset limit. My grandfather, or any other patient of the time, would not be able to take advantage of this advance as the electronic pacemaker had not yet been invented. So he was a laboratory for the natural course of this disease, which was to get a progressively slower and slower heart rate making him prone to syncope, know as Stokes-Adams attacks. This is a sudden loss of consciousness because of a heart rate that has gotten too slow. My grandmother would hear a thump on the floor, know immediately what happened, and find my grandfather lying unconscious. Slowly his ventricles would speed up enough for him to regain consciousness. When I was eighteen years old, and a freshman in college, my grandfather collapsed in the bathroom. I heard the thump and ran in. He was completely unconscious and I thought he was dead. I picked him off the floor and carried him to the bedroom and placed him on his back on the bed. I took his pulse and I felt nothing. I was about to tell my grandmother the bad news when I suddenly felt a pulse beat, so I kept on palpating his radial pulse and after what seemed like an eternity I felt another heart beat. I kept counting and I felt one heart beat every six seconds for a heart rate of ten beats per minute. Finally it slowly sped up, and he regained consciousness. In all the years I have practiced medicine, I never had a patient with a heart beat as slow as when I was eighteen years old and had my first cardiac examination experience. He died of his problem six months later when I was back at school.

A fifty-six year old woman was seen with a chief complaint of shortness of breath, especially with exertion. More recently she also complained of suddenly being awakened from sleep very short of breath. This is known as paroxysmal nocturnal dyspnea and can be caused by left-sided heart failure. Examination of her heart revealed a softly blowing systolic murmur, and what I interpreted as a gallop rhythm. The murmur was maximal in intensity near the apex (bottom) of the heart and suggested the diagnosis of mitral insufficiency. In other words, the mitral valve between the left atrium and the left ventricle did not close completely when her ventricle beat, therefore some of the blood ejected from the left ventricle, instead of going to the aorta through the aortic valve, leaked back through the incompletely closed mitral valve into the left atrium. There are a number of causes for this including an enlarged left ventricle and rheumatic fever. But I didn't expect to find what the echocardiogram identified—a left atrial myxoma, a benign and rare cardiac tumor. Surgery was curative.

PULMONARY

Inspection: During the cardiac examination, your anterior chest wall was carefully inspected. Now your physician will inspect your posterior, or the back side of your chest. He will first look for symmetry. Are both sides equal in appearance? Your breathing will be noted, taking into account how both sides of your chest rise as you inhale. If they do not expand equally you may have a rib injury, lung collapse, pneumonia, or pleurisy—an inflammation of the outer lining of your lung. The anterior-posterior (front to back) diameter should be less than the side to side diameter. If they are equal this could mean you have emphysema (progressive collapse of the air sacs of your lungs). In this condition, your inspection may reveal large neck muscles caused by their constant over use in helping you breathe.

Palpation: Your physician can touch your chest with the palm of his hand. At the same time you are asked to repeat the words "ninety-nine." When you do so, he will feel vibrations, and these vibrations—known as tactile fremitus—should be equal on both sides of your chest.

Reduced or absent tactile fremitus can occur when you have a collapsed lung, fluid in your chest cavity, thickening of the lining of your lung (pleura), or obstructed bronchial tubes.

An increased fremitus can result when the lung has consolidated (hardened or compressed) as can occur with some pneumonias.

Percussion: A normal lung will give a typical note when your chest is percussed. This note should be similar on both sides of the chest.

If the note is louder or more resonant, it suggests that there is more air under the percussing fingers than normal. This can clinch the diagnosis of an injured lung where air has escaped into the chest cage (pneumothorax), or emphysema where the lung is over inflated due to the damaged air sacs.

If the note is duller than usual, it could men that you have pneumonia, collapsed lung, fluid in your chest cavity, or tumor.

Your physician can also determine if your diaphragm moves down when you breathe in and up when you breathe out. The diaphragm separates the lungs from the abdominal contents. You will be asked to "exhale completely and hold it."

Then your physician may percuss your lungs on both sides and will mark off the upper limit of your diaphragm. He will do it again after asking you to "inhale completely and hold it." This inhalation will lower your diaphragm and allow your physician to mark off the diaphragm's lower limits. Normally the diaphragmatic motion should be three to seven centimeters depending upon your physical conditioning.

The failure of your diaphragm to move with breathing could be due either to lung pathology, such as a lung mass or lung collapse—or intraabdominal pathology such as a liver mass.

Auscultation: When your physician uses a stethoscope and listens to your lungs while you deeply breathe through your mouth, he is listening for breath sounds. There are many variations of breath sounds, but in essence the sound is either increased or decreased.

Decreased breath sounds occur when your breaths are prevented from reaching your physician's ear. This may occur if your bronchial tree is obstructed by a mucus plug or a foreign body. Decreased breath sounds also occur in emphysema when the lungs sacs (alveoli) have collapsed and coalesced so that the lungs are hyperinflated and air moves poorly; if your pleura is thickened, thus preventing the air from reaching the stethoscope; if your lung has collapsed; or if you have pneumonia.

Increased breath sounds can occur when pneumonia has become severe enough to consolidate or compress your lung. When your breath travels down your bronchial tree and hits this consolidated patch, it will enhance the transmission of the sound to the stethoscope.

If your physician hears cellophane like crackles in your lungs it could mean either a pneumonia or congestive heart failure due to fluid accumulation.

If wheezes on expiration are heard, you may have bronchial asthma or congestive heart failure.

The above mentioned examinations performed on the posterior chest should also be performed on the anterior chest.

CLINICAL EXAMPLES

As an intern I admitted a patient to the hospital for fever, weight loss, night sweats and a chronic productive cough. Our initial presumptive diagnosis was tuberculosis. On the day of admission an elderly attending physician came to Cook County to make rounds with us. This physician had an excellent reputation as an outstanding diagnostician. We eagerly looked forward to his visits. It seemed to us that there was absolutely nothing that this man did not know, and he was a superb teacher. He had been practicing almost fifty years, and was trained in the early twentieth century including a few years in Vienna—if memory serves me correctly—at the Allgemiene Krankenhaus. Rumor had it he would wake up every morning at five o'clock to study the latest medical literature. It was the custom to present each case by giving the full medical history, which we provided to this esteemed physician. He looked at the patient carefully, and asked him to sit up in bed with legs over the side. The physician then took up position facing the patient's back and proceeded to percuss his lung fields. This seemed to take an unusual amount of time, and when he finished, he said to us, "Come closer and bring a pen." We did. "Listen carefully," he said, and he percussed slowly and every few seconds he would stop and make a mark on the patient's skin. We listened and watched as he percussed from right to left and left to right, from up to down and down to up. When he finished he had a clearly defined ten by twelve centimeter oval marked out on the patient's posterior, upper chest. He said, "I agree with your diagnosis of tuberculosis, but I think you'll also find that this patient has a tubercular lung abscess located here." We all looked at each other in amazement, for this was a remarkable achievement, not likely equaled by anyone else in that room—or any room for that matter. An X-ray of the chest confirmed the abscess precisely where the physician had percussed it out on the patient's chest. This physician was trained when William Konrad Roentgen discovered X-rays. Physicians trained in that era had nothing to go on except their own senses, so they developed them to a physical diagnostic capability we will probably never equal in the modern high-tech physician.

A young man came to Cook County Hospital complaining of shortness of breath. Examination of the lungs demonstrated the following on the right side: observation—absent respiratory movement; palpation—no findings; percussion—loud, hollow sound; tactile fremitus—absent; auscultation—no breath sounds. This man had the classical findings of a pneumothorax (air in the chest cavity caused by a ruptured lung allowing air to escape from the air sacs into the chest cavity). The air pressure in the chest cavity results in a lung collapse—either partial or complete. Pneumothorax results most commonly from trauma, but there was no history of same in this case. He had what is known a spontaneous pneumothorax, caused by a ruptured air cyst on the lung. This is one of the easier diagnoses to make based on physical examination findings. An x-ray was taken, confirmed the diagnosis, and told us the extent of the pneumothorax.

GASTROINTESTINAL

As mentioned in the history, if you draw two lines on your abdomen straight down and across through your umbilicus (belly button) you will have divided your abdomen into four equal quadrants: your right upper quadrant; left upper quadrant; right lower quadrant; left lower quadrant. These landmarks make it possible for your physician to accurately place abdominal findings discovered during the course of the physical examination.

Inspection: Your physician will have you lie flat so as best to inspect your abdomen. By bringing his eyes at eye level to your abdomen from your side, he will be able to roughly evaluate your nutritional status. Also a careful observation of your abdomen could reveal the presence of an enlarged liver or spleen, or a hernia, or an abnormal pulsation due to an aortic aneurysm. A careful look at your umbilicus could also present your physician with important clues: it might be inverted with the presence of an intraabdominal mass or fluid in the belly (ascites); it will be significantly everted (protruberant) with an umbilical hernia; red and tender if it is inflamed; or if there is intrabdominal bleeding, the skin around the umbilicus may be blue (Cullen's sign).

Auscultation: We will discuss auscultation next because when you palpate or percuss the abdomen you may uncover tenderness and increase intestinal motion (peristalsis), possibly resulting in an erroneous impression of the bowel sounds as heard via the stethoscope. Bowel sounds are caused by the movement of air and food or liquids through the intestines. They have a characteristic sound that is considered normal, and this sound should be heard on an average of eight to ten times per minute. If they are high-pitched and tinkling, it could mean an intestinal obstruction. If they are absent (after listening for a full five minutes), it suggests intestinal paralysis (ileus).

The other reason to listen to the abdomen is the possibility of hearing a bruit. Normally such sounds would be absent. If they are heard it speaks to an obstruction of an abdominal artery or an aneurysm of an artery.

Percussion: What can your physician learn by careful percussion of your abdomen? He can evaluate your liver size by percussing your lower right chest and right upper quadrant of the abdomen. The same thing can be done to determine your spleen size by percussing your left upper quadrant. By percussion and proper positioning it is also possible to determine if there is any fluid within your abdominal cavity. Mostly percussion of the abdomen, which is not completely reliable, has been replaced by various imaging studies of the abdomen, but a careful examination can raise strong suspicions that will need to be confirmed or denied.

Palpation: To undergo a successful palpation of your abdomen you must be lying flat on your back, preferably with your knees bent. This has the effect of relaxing your abdominal wall, allowing deeper palpation thus making your physician's palpatory efforts more reliable. With proper positioning it is possible to easily palpate an enlarged liver or spleen. It is even possible to palpate an enlarged kidney. Obesity negates the effectiveness of abdominal palpation.

Tenderness in any of the abdominal quadrants can indicate inflammation: appendicitis—right lower quadrant; inflamed colon pockets (diverticulitis)—left lower quadrant; inflamed gall bladder (cholecystitis)—right upper quadrant; pancreatitis—left upper quadrant or upper middle of abdomen.

If your abdomen is tender your physician may want to test you for rebound tenderness. He will press the tips of his fingers deeply—and suddenly let go. If you experience severe pain when he suddenly lets go it is known as rebound tenderness. This is a serious sign that could indicate peritonitis. This test should be reserved for the last part of the abdominal examination, because it can be very painful, and you will be less likely to stay relaxed.

I will include the rectal examination in this section.

Inspection: Your physician will perform a visual inspection of your anal area to see if there is any inflammation, splits in the skin—fissure, drainage near the anal opening—fistula, evidence of hemmorhoids (dilated veins), or skin irritation due to pruritis ani. While inspecting he may ask you to bear down to determine if there is any prolapse, or protrusion out through the anal opening of rectal mucosa (lining) or hemorrhoids.

Inflammation or tenderness or a dimple above the anus and below the coccyx indicates the presence of a pilonoidal cyst. This is a congenital condition: a sinus (passageway), which may get infected and drain pus. Surgery is necessary for a complete cure

Palpation: With a well lubricated rectal glove your physician will perform a digital rectal examination. The first thing he will determine is if your rectal muscular sphincter is tight and not lax. The latter could be seen in neurological disorders. The principle reason to do a digital rectal examination is to make certain there is no rectal mass (cancer) present. In the male your physician will carefully evaluate your prostate (see Genitourinary section of the physical exam).

CLINICAL EXAMPLES

A middle aged man developed sudden onset of severe abdominal pain. In order to walk he had to stoop forward and clutch his abdomen. He had never experienced such intense pain before. His physical examination demonstrated marked left lower quadrant tenderness, including rebound tenderness. When he lay on his back he kept his knees up, which helped relieve some of the discomfort he was experiencing. His abdomen was distended, and bowel sounds were greatly diminished. A rectal examination was uncomfortable for the patient, but there was no blood or any masses palpable. He had a low grade fever and an elevated white blood cell count. An x-ray of the abdomen showed air under the diaphragm. This meant that the patient experienced a gastrointestinal tract perforation with the escape of air into the abdominal cavity. The location of the positive abdominal tenderness suggested the possibility of a perforation of a colon diverticulum (outpouching of the colon), or a perforated malignancy. Surgery was performed, a ruptured diverticulum was found and a short segment of the colon was resected. The patient did well postoperatively.

A diabetic patient was under good control taking oral diabetic medication. He watched his diet carefully, had lost twenty pounds and was doing well. I saw him every three months on follow up visits. On one occasion he came to the office at his wife's insistence, because she thought the whites of his eyes had turned yellow. She was correct. Not only his eyes, but his skin was also developing a yellow tinge. A urinalysis demonstrated dark urine and a rectal examination showed light colored stool on the examining finger. Clearly the patient had developed what is known as obstructive jaundice. Something was blocking the entry of bile into the intestines. He had no pain whatsoever. This is known as silent jaundice, and one of the main causes is cancer of the pancreas, which this patient was proven to have. Unfortunately, it was inoperable. He knew precisely what lie in store for him, and he chose to quickly put all his affairs in order. To do this gave him great comfort in what was to be his remaining few weeks.

GENITOURINARY

I will discuss the examination of the male genitourinary system in this section. The examination of the female genitourinary system will be discussed under gynecology.

The penis is examined first. It is observed and palpated by your physician's gloved fingers. He is looking for any penile lesions. The opening of your urethra should be at the very end of the penile shaft, and be clear of discharge. If a discharge is found, it should be collected for bacterial culture and microscopic examination.

Examination of the scrotum and testes is next. Using both gloved hands your physician will palpate your testicles and other intrascrotal contents. It will be a simple matter for him to identify a testicular mass (infection or tumor), absence of a testicle, shrunken testicles, a hernia, a varicocele (dilated veins—which feels like a 'bag of worms'), epididymitis (an infection of the epididymis—a tube that delivers sperm into the urethra). If your physician is unsure as to whether a mass is fluid or a solid tumor, he can shine a light through your scrotum. Fluid transilluminates (shows as a red glow). A solid tumor does not.

Your physician will perform a prostate examination by inserting his index finger into your rectum. The prostate is easily evaluated for: enlargements, which may be benign or malignant; tenderness, which suggests infection; and hard nodules or asymmetric enlargement of one of the prostate lobes, both of which suggests a fifty percent chance of cancer.

CLINICAL EXAMPLES

A patient of mine brought her sixty-eight year old husband to see me. He was complaining of severe back pain and had been diagnosed as having Paget's disease. This is a disorder of bone where the normal turnover of bone (old bone cells being replaced by new) is accelerated in certain localized areas. The normal bone matrix is replaced with softened and enlarged bone. The x-ray picture shows increased bone whiteness, coarseness and thickening. In spite of symptomatic attempts at pain relief, his pain worsened. I examined the patient, and the main physical finding was discovered on his rectal examination. His prostate gland was enlarged, irregular and hard. It was filled with several easily palpable, rock hard, one to two centimeter nodules. This was diagnostic for prostate cancer and was confirmed with a prostate specific antigen test of over two thousand (the highest I had ever seen). The normal prostate specific antigen test is under four (although one could have cancer even with a normal PSA). This patient had advanced prostate cancer with metastasis to the bone (paget's disease can mimic this x-ray picture). He underwent orchiectomy (removal of the testicles), and was referred to an oncologist for chemotherapy. He had instant relief lasting for two years until the disease reasserted itself and spread to his liver.

A sixty year old woman was seen in follow up for hypertension. As part of the physical examination, I thought I could palpate a mass in the patient's right upper abdominal quadrant under the liver. I ordered a CT scan of the abdomen and it showed a very large kidney cyst. Since she was asymptomatic, and the cyst did not demonstrate any CT findings suggesting malignancy, it was left alone, but it is being followed with scans that can determine if there are any changes suggesting a trend toward malignant degeneration.

GYNECOLOGICAL

You will be placed in the lithotomy position for a gynecological examination. You will be positioned lying on your back on the examining table with your feet in stirrups, knees apart and buttocks at the end of the table. Your urinary bladder should be emptied before the examination.

The first part of the examination is an external evaluation. Your physician will observe for any deviations from normal exterior anatomy including your urethra (opening of the urinary bladder).

The internal vaginal examination is performed using a speculum, which allows for complete examination of the vagina and cervix. With the speculum in place, a PAP smear of your cervix can be performed.

A bimanual examination is also done. One of your physician's hands will be placed on your lower abdomen and the other inserted in your vagina. This allows examination of your uterus, ovaries and fallopian tubes. It is possible to determine if there are any tumors of these organs, or if there is evidence of infection (severe tenderness or discharge).

A combined rectovaginal examination with one finger in the rectum and another in the vagina allows your physician to evaluate your rectum and rectovaginal septum—the thick layer of tissue separating these two organs.

CLINICAL EXAMPLES

When I completed my internship at Cook County Hospital there was no chance to start a residency, because there was a doctor draft in place and we were all committed to spend two years in the military. This was a known and expected interlude to what already was a long educational experience. We spent six weeks training at Fort Sam Houston, Texas, and then received our duty assignment. I and my new bride were assigned to the 101st airborne division at Fort Campbell, Kentucky. During our orientation, the chief of service, an obstetrician, asked his new medical recruits, "Who among you have delivered babies?" Four of us raised our hands. "How many?" he asked. Since my volume was two hundred deliveries more than my closest competitor, the chief, a lieutenant colonel, said, "Okay

Captain Cohen, you're on OB call. You'll work with me today and start call tomorrow." Like any good soldier, all I could say was "Yes sir." In the time spent at Fort Campbell, I added a considerable number of deliveries to my total, and I also learned an important lesson that I have never forgotten. I saw a young lady in the gynecology clinic who complained of pelvic pain. The pain was sudden in onset and accompanied by some vaginal spotting. Her vital signs were unremarkable. I performed a pelvic examination and found her to have tenderness and pain when her cervix was moved. My initial impression was pelvic inflammatory disease (PID), a diagnosis made many times at Cook County Hospital. I told the commander about the case and my diagnosis. He said, "Did she miss any periods?" "Uhh—I forgot to ask," I weakly answered. He asked the patient, and she had. He examined her and turned to me and said, "This lady has an ectopic pregnancy." She went promptly to surgery. Yes, my chief was right. This was a humbling and important lesson for me, something that I'm sure all physicians experience more than one time or another during their careers.

My time spent at Fort Campbell was most interesting and educational. My wife worked as a Red Cross nurse giving various immunizations to the "tough paratroopers," as she described them. "Some of them fainted when they saw my needle." We often saw the paratroopers do their required jumps, and as we watched them float gracefully to the ground, I said to my wife, "Isn't that great, I'm going to do that one of these days." "Yeah, right," she chuckled. "I can just see you doing that." Well, she did—fifty years later. In celebration of my seventy-fifth birthday, I sky dived from 14,000 feet (tandem jump). And those paratroopers only jumped from a thousand!

A patient was seen in the office of a classmate of mine. Her chief complaint was a vaginal discharge. My friend, a family practitioner who was brand new in practice, examined the patient and confirmed the presence of a purulent vaginal discharge. On speculum examination he discovered the cause—a foreign body was present, and this set up the infection. The foreign body turned out to be a condom. Now the rest of this story should have never happened, but it did, and probably speaks to inexperience. Apparently my friend jokingly reassured the patient's husband that his wife had developed an infection because of a foreign body left in her vagina, and that they both needed to be more careful and make sure that the condom is not forgotten in the heat of passion. The husband's response—"Doctor, I don't use condoms."

MUSCULOSKELETAL

The musculoskeletal system consists of three parts: bones, joints and muscles. There are 206 bones in the human body, and the joints are either synovial or nonsynovial. Synovial joints are freely movable, have bones that are separated and enclosed in a joint cavity that is filled with a lubricating fluid called synovial fluid. This fluid, plus cartilage on the ends of the bones, allows the opposing bones to slide over each other. Ligaments stretch from bone to bone and strengthen the joints. Bursa are sacs filled with fluid and are located in areas where friction may result. Bursa help muscles and ligaments and tendons glide smoothly over bones.

Synovial joints include fingers, toes, wrists, ankles, elbows, knees, hips, shoulders and the temperomandibular joints. The latter permits jaw movement for speaking and chewing. Nonsynovial joints are found in the spine.

Your physician will inspect and palpate your joints looking for masses, deformity, redness, tenderness and swelling. A swollen joint could be due to fluid accumulation in the joint, or thickening of the synovial lining as seen in various forms of arthritis.

Your joints are evaluated for range of motion to determine of there are limitations. Limitation of motion may be due to infection, trauma, or arthritis.

Each joint has characteristic methods of examination that can determine range of motion as well as muscle strength. There are special examinations for the spine and legs that could raise suspicion for a herniated (slipped) disc.

CLINICAL EXAMPLES

On a routine follow-up examination of a fifty-four year old female diabetic patient, I was told that she was experiencing dull and aching pain in her right shoulder. She also said that the movement of her shoulder was becoming more difficult as time went on. She had some localized tenderness along the upper shoulder and upper arm. Her range of motion, was clearly limited. She could not remember any recent trauma to her shoulder. I wasn't sure why she was having this difficulty, but I recommended she see an orthopedic surgeon. The orthopedist made a diagnosis of "frozen shoulder." Why it happens, no one is sure, but it does occur more frequently in diabetics. The capsule of the shoulder gets inflamed and thickened and freezes up. He prescribed anti-inflammatory medications, heat and physical therapy including stretching and range of motion exercises. He reserved the use of cortisone injections if this initial therapy wasn't enough. The illness does get better in time.

As an intern at Cook County Hospital I saw a young man in the orthopedic clinic who had injured his right arm. Physical examination revealed a deformity of his right humerus. It was severely swollen, black and blue and very tender. The deformity was located about six inches down from the top of his shoulder. An x-ray revealed a complete break with the bone separated and angled at the fracture line. The orthopedist told me to put on a hanging arm cast with a sling. This is a cast from the shoulder to the wrist with the elbow bent at a right angle. The theory is that the heavy cast pulls the bone into place and it will gradually heal. The patient was given post-cast instructions and told to return to the clinic in three weeks. He did as he was told and when I saw him in three weeks he seemed fine except for one thing—he wasn't wearing a cast! "What happened to the cast?" I asked. "When I left here last time I had to play a basketball game, so I cut off the cast," he answered. Amazed, I asked, "Did you put it back on?" "No," he smiled. I shook my head in disbelief. An x-ray showed perfect healing with a straight humerus and solid callous (new bone).

Mother Nature is still the best healer!

NEUROLOGICAL

Anatomy: A carefully performed neurological examination may provide your physician with accurate information in terms of localization of an abnormality to a specific neurological site. We will go through the examination of the various parts of the nervous system, but first—a general and brief discussion of the anatomy and physiology.

The nervous system is divided into two parts: central nervous system and peripheral nervous system.

The central nervous system includes the spinal cord and the brain.

The peripheral nervous system includes:

1. Twelve pairs of cranial nerves that originate in the brain. They direct muscular movements of the head and neck and receive sensations from the head and neck;

2. Thirty-one spinal nerves that control body and extremity muscular movement, and receive sensations from the periphery to the spinal cord and ultimately up to the brain.

The brain's outer layer is called the cerebral cortex. The cortex is divided into two halves: right and left—known as the right cerebral hemisphere, and the left cerebral hemisphere. The cerebral cortex is the sight of your intellect. It is responsible for insight, thought, memory and reasoning. Both cerebral hemispheres have four lobes, each responsible for specific functions. These are:

1. Frontal lobe—personality, intellect and emotions.

2. Parietal lobe—sensation.

3. Occipital lobe—sight.

4. Temporal lobe—hearing and speech.

The cerebellum is another part of the brain, separate and below the cerebral cortex. It is responsible for coordinating complex muscular movements (running, walking, swimming, playing a musical instrument). The cerebellum operates automatically—under the conscious level.

The basal ganglia are nerve bands buried deep within both cerebral hemispheres. They control automatic associated body movements.

The thalamus acts as a relay station between the spine and the cerebral cortex where neurons (nerve cells) meet (synapse). This relay station delivers impulses to the periphery from the brain and to the brain from the periphery.

The brain stem is a connecting nerve link from the spinal cord to the brain. It is made up of three parts where nerve tracts ascend and descend. It is also responsible for automatic control of respiration, heart and gastrointestinal function.

The spinal cord occupies the upper seventy percent of the bony vertebral canal. It consists of long nerve tracts that start in the periphery (skin, muscles, tendons, internal organs), enter your spinal cord and finally your brain. These nerve tracts deliver sensations: temperature (hot, cold), touch, pain, vibration—to your brain (sensory pathways). Also these nerve tracts deliver messages from the brain to the periphery that control purposeful movements (motor pathways).

Neurological examination:

Motor: Basically the motor examination has already been done. This portion of the neurological examination is to assess your muscular function. Are your movements well coordinated, or do they exhibit rigidity and spasticity, or show wasting (atrophy). Your physician may have you take a short walk back and forth in the examining room, or up and down the hallway. He may ask you to walk a straight line going heel to toe. In this way he can assess your motor power, control and gait. Evaluation of your gait can give valuable clues to neurological disorders:

A staggering, wide based gait with turning difficulty and poorly coordinated movement could mean cerebellar disease such as alcohol induced cerebellar damage, cerebellar tumor, or multiple sclerosis.

A stooped posture with flexed knees, hips and elbows, short, shuffling steps, absence of arm swings and a mask like face is diagnostic of Parkinson's disease.

Cranial nerves: Your cranial nerves can be tested individually.

Cranial Nerve I—Olfactory nerve. This nerve gives you your sense of smell. Decreased sense of smell can be caused by allergies, tobacco, sinusitis, upper respiratory infection and cocaine. Any lesion in the brain that involves the olfactory nerve could destroy your sense of smell (anosmia). Ordinarily this is not tested unless you report a distinct loss. Your physician can use coffee, vanilla, pepper, toothpaste, or any other non-irritating substance. Each nostril should be tested separately, and a distinct difference in the two sides is significant.

Cranial Nerve II—Optic nerve. This nerve gives you sight. The optic nerve can be directly visualized on your retinas with the use of an ophthalmoscope. A swelling and blurring of the optic nerve head (papilledema) is indicative of increased intracranial pressure seen with a brain tumor. Optic atrophy (which can eventually cause blindness) can also be identified as a gradual destruction of the optic nerve. The causes include: optic neuritis, a degenerative disease of unknown cause, although an occasional patient with optic neuritis will develop multiple sclerosis; other cases of optic neuritis include glaucoma, blood vessel disorders, nutritional deficiency, poisons, untreated syphilis and a brain tumor. There is a hereditary form known as Leber's hereditary optic atrophy.

Cranial Nerve III, IV, VI—Occulomotor, Trochlear, Abducens nerves. These nerves control your eye movements by innervating the extraoccular muscles (small muscles attached to your eyeballs). They also control your pupil size and eyelids. Dysfunction of one or more of these nerves can also cause ptosis (drooping of an eyelid), or inability to turn your eyeball in a specific direction. Your physician may assess this function by standing in front of you and asking you to 'hold your head still and keep your eyes focused on my finger as I move it.'

Cranial Nerve V—Trigeminal nerve. This nerve controls your chewing muscles, and carries sensory input from your face. For the motor portion of the exam your physician will touch your jaws and ask you to chew. He should feel firm movement of your jaw muscles on both sides of your face. For the sensory portion he will ask you to close your eyes, touch your face lightly—perhaps with a wisp of cotton—and ask if you feel it by saying the word 'now.' He will do this on the upper middle and lower portion of your face to assess the function of the three branches of the nerve: ophthalmic, maxillary and mandibular.

Cranial Nerve VII—Facial nerve. This nerve innervates the muscles of the face. It is a simple matter to ask you to smile, talk, whistle, wrinkle your forehead and frown. If you can do all these easily your nerve is working well on both sides of your face.

The sensory function of this nerve provides you with a sense of taste. If you complain of a loss of taste, it can easily be tested by placing sugar or salt or lemon juice on your tongue and ask you to identify.

If your physician touches your cornea with a wisp of cotton, he is testing your corneal reflex. The normal reflex is to blink. If you do not, you could have a lesion in cranial nerve V, (sensory fibers) or cranial nerve VII (motor fibers).

Cranial Nerve VIII—Acoustic nerve also called Vestibulocochlear nerve. This is the nerve of hearing and balance.

Cranial Nerve IX and X. Glossopharyngeal and Vagus nerve. The glossopharyngeal nerve controls movement of the tongue, uvula and soft palate. This can be assessed by the use of a tongue blade pressed on your tongue and watching your uvula, soft palate and tonsillar pillars move.

The vagus nerve is the only nerve that originates in the brainstem and extends all the way to the abdomen. It is considered the most important nerve in the body. It supplies fibers to all the organs except the adrenal glands. It functions automatically, controlling your heart beat, muscles of the larynx (speech) and gastrointestinal organs down to the transverse colon. You have no conscious control of your vagus (except for the few larynx muscles), and your physician cannot test its automatic function.

Cranial Nerve XI—Spinal Accessory nerve. This nerve controls head rotation and shoulder movement. Your physician will examine this function by asking you to turn your head against the resistance of his hand on your face, and asking you to shrug your shoulders while he attempts to prevent this movement. Your movements should be equally strong on both sides.

Cranial Nerve XII—Hypoglossal Nerve. This nerve innervates the tongue. You should have good control of its movements and be able to speak. Your physician may ask you to say words starting with the letters l, t, d, and n where the tongue is used to form the words. They should be clear and distinct.

Cerebellar function

Romberg test: This test was described under the vestibular system. You will be asked to stand with feet together, hands at your sides and eyes closed. An abnormal test is swaying and a loss of balance worse when eyes are closed. In addition to evaluating your ear's balance mechanism, this test also is positive with cerebellar dysfunction.

Another test for cerebellar dysfunction is rapid alternating movements. You will be asked to pat your knees with both the front and back of your hands in rapid succession. You should be able to do this in a coordinated manner. A slow, clumsy, uncoordinated response suggests a cerebellar disorder.

Finger to finger test is performed as follows: Your physician will ask you to place your index finger on your nose. He will hold his finger in front of your face about two feet away. He will then ask you to touch his moving finger with your finger and then touch your nose. A normal response is a rapid finger to nose back and forth coordinated movement.

There is another finger to nose test where your physician asks you to hold both hands out to your sides, and then rapidly (with eyes closed) alternately touch your index finger to your nose as rapidly as possible. An abnormal test would be a completely uncoordinated attempt to touch your nose.

The last test for cerebellar dysfunction is to lie flat on your back, place one heel on the opposite knee and slowly run your heel down your shin. Normally this can be done easily. In an abnormal test your heel will fall off your shin.

Sensory tests: The sensations tested include light touch, pain, temperature, vibration and position.

Light touch is tested by touching you on both sides of your body with a wisp of cotton while your eyes are closed. You will be asked to say "touch" each time you feel the cotton.

Pain is tested by your physician touching your body with the sharp end of a pin or the dull end. You will be asked to say "sharp" or "dull" whenever you feel yourself being touched.

To test temperature discrimination your physician will touch your body with a hot and cold object and ask that you say "hot" or "cold."

These three sensations—light touch, pain and temperature travel through the peripheral nerve through the spinal cord in a tract known as the spinothalamic tract and finally up to the cerebral cortex where the sensation is felt.

Failure to pass one of these tests could indicate an abnormality either of the peripheral nerves involved, the spinothalamic tract in the spinal cord, or the cerebral cortex.

Vibration sense is tested by your physician holding a vibrating tuning fork over the bony prominences of your wrists and shin bones. You should easily feel the vibrations equally on both sides.

If your physician grabs your toe and moves it up or down, you should be able to easily tell (without looking) which direction your toe is moved. This is called position sense (kinesthesia).

If your physician places a coin or key in your hand, you should be able to identify the object by feel alone. This is called stereognosis.

Your physician may trace a number on the palm of your hand with your eyes closed. You should be able to identify the number. This is called graphesthesia.

These sensations—vibration, kinesthesia and graphesthesia travel through the peripheral nerve through the spinal cord in a tract known as the posterior column tract and finally up to the cerebral cortex where the sensation is felt.

Reflexes: You are familiar with reflexes (the typical knee jerk when the knee is struck with a reflex hammer). A reflex is a mechanism that operates below the level of consciousness. It permits a quick response to a potentially dangerous situation. As an example when the knee is struck, the sensation travels through the peripheral nerve to the spinal cord where the sensation meets another nerve tract, which sends an impulse to the muscle ordering your leg to 'jerk'. This is called a reflex arc.

Your physician will test for a number of different deep tendon reflexes. These include:

Biceps reflex: The biceps tendon is struck. This arc travels through cervical vertebrae C5 to C6.

Triceps reflex: The triceps tendon is struck. This arc travels through cervical vertebrae C7 to C8.

Brachioradialis reflex: The forearm tendon is struck. This arc travels through cervical vertebrae C5 to C6.

Quadriceps reflex: The knee is struck ('knee jerk'). This arc travels through lumbar (lower back vertebrae) L2 to L4.

Achilles reflex: The Achilles tendon is struck (ankle jerk). This arc travels through lumbar and sacral vertebrae (L5 to S2).

Your physician will grade your reflexes on a four point scale:

4+ very brisk. Usually indicates pathology.

3+ brisker than average. May indicate pathology.

2+ Normal

1+ Lower than normal. Diminished response

0 No response. May be abnormal.

Your reflexes should be equal on the right and left side. A difference is usually abnormal.

An abnormal reflex suggests some pathology somewhere along the reflex arc from the periphery to the spinal cord and back to the periphery.

Besides the above stretch reflexes there are also superficial reflexes:

Abdominal—your abdominal skin is touched from the lateral side toward the midline on both upper quadrants and both lower quadrants. A normal response is an abdominal muscle contraction. This reflex is absent with diseases of the spinal cord's pyramidal tract, and is also absent on the opposite side of a cerebral vascular accident (stroke).

Plantar reflex—Babinski's reflex or extensor plantar reflex. This is a very important reflex. Your physician will stroke the outer aspect of the sole of your foot from the heel to your toes. An abnormal response is when the great toe flexes toward the top of your foot and the other toes fan out. In infants and young children to age two this response is considered normal. After age two (when the neurological system has fully developed) it is considered abnormal. The presence of this abnormal reflex indicates damage to the nerve tracts connecting the spinal cord to the brain. If you have this abnormal reflex, it brings to your physician's mind a long list of diagnoses including spinal cord disease, cerebellar tumor, stroke, head injury, meningitis, autoimmune neurological disorders such as multiple sclerosis, amyotrophic lateral sclerosis (Lou Gehrig's disease) and brain involvement from liver failure.

CLINICAL EXAMPLES

During my intern days at Cook County Hospital I spent a month on the neurology service. There were a number of patients who lived on the ward. They had unusual neurological symptoms and physical findings, and in return for being boarded they served as teaching examples for medical students and interns and residents. One cooperative patient had a classical syndrome. His neurological examination revealed findings mostly localized to the lower extremities. His lower legs were atonic (weak muscles). Patellar and Achilles tendon reflexes were absent. He could not feel a vibrating tuning fork touching his shins. When you moved his toes up or down with his eyes closed, he did not know in which direction you moved them. He failed the heel to knee test. He did not feel pinpricks on his legs and his Romberg sign was positive. When he stood upright with his eyes open he had no trouble standing, but when he closed his eyes, he would instantly lose his balance. Ordinarily we can stand with our eyes closed and not lose our balance, because we can feel sensations from the bottom of our feet and know where we are. We also know where we are because of our vision. In the case of this patient, he lost the ability to know where he was based upon the pathology of his legs and feet, but he could keep his balance if his eyes were open. When he closed his eyes, however, he lost both mechanisms (eye and feet), and since he had nothing to tell him where he was, he would quickly lose his balance. With all these abnormal neurological findings, it was clear that this patient lost the use of the posterior columns in his spinal cord. And he lost them because they were destroyed by syphilis in a condition known as tabes dorsalis, which manifests itself about twenty to thirty years after the initial infection.

A "droopy eyelid" was the chief complaint of a middle aged man who came to my office. A droopy eyelid is termed ptosis. On examination, his right eyelid was closed and he could not raise it by willing himself to do so. I examined him and found that the pupil on the same side was miotic (tiny) compared to the left. Clinically, it was clear that the patient had ptosis and miosis on the right. This is two thirds of a triad of symptoms, the third one being absence of sweating of the face on the same side (anhidrosis). I asked him if he noticed this symptom, but he wasn't sure. If I remember correctly, I saw him during the winter months. Anyhow, the neurological findings of ptosis, miosis and anhidrosis is a characteristic triad known as Horner's syndrome—caused by an interruption of the autonomic sympathetic nerve supply to the eye. This interruption can be caused by a stroke in various parts of the brain or by a tumor on the very top of the lung (apex) known as a pancoast tumor. Because the patient had been a smoker for many years, this was my first impression. Unfortunately it was confirmed by a chest x-ray.

You have completed the physical examination. Your physician now has more data to add to the history. He may have clinched a diagnosis, or increased his level of suspicion in one direction or the other. He will now take this enhanced data base and see what the laboratory studies add.

PART III
LABORATORY DATA

✦

*"All things are to be examined and
called into question.
There are no limits set to thought."*

Edith Hamilton
(1867–1963)

INTRODUCTION

An important part of your complete physical examination is a screening laboratory analysis. It provides vital information that when taken together with your history and physical examination will allow your physician to diagnose you with a high degree of certainty. The need for more specific studies—apart from the screening laboratory data—can be ordered if necessary.

I will first provide a brief description of the test and its clinical significance. I will follow the description of each test with two sections: ELEVATION and REDUCTION. The lists will not be all-inclusive, nor will it include detailed discussion. The interested patient can utilize the internet (Google for instance) and find answers with a click of the finger.

The complete screening analysis includes:

COMPLETE BLOOD COUNT MEASURING THREE DIFFERENT TYPES OF CELLS

1. White blood cells.

These members of your immune surveillance system protect your body against bacteria, viruses, fungi and parasites. When we are confronted by one of these organisms, a chemical message causes the bone marrow to produce more white blood cells that rush to attack and destroy the invaders. White blood cells also protect your body against any cells that they identify as foreign, such as cancer cells. The body also identifies a transplanted organ as foreign, and launches an attack against it. That is why anti-rejection medications must be used. When this immune surveillance mechanism goes awry, and the white blood cells mistakenly attack normal tissue, an autoimmune illness may result. There are five different types of white blood cells. Each type plays a distinct role in the body's surveillance against infection. The rise in the number count of the individual type of white cell gives a clue as to the identification of the invader.

Your complete blood count report will include the total white blood cell count as well as the total count of each of the five different white cells (differential count). The normal total white blood count is five to ten thousand.

ELEVATION

Stress (physical or emotional)
Infection (bacterial, viral, fungal, parasitic)
Leukemia (acute or chronic)
Bone marrow disease (myeloproliferative disorder)
Medications (cortisone, antiseizure drugs, antibiotics)
Burns or other injuries causing tissue damage

REDUCTION

Viral infections including HIV
Medications (chemotherapy, antibiotics and many common medications)
Radiation therapy
Leukemia
Bone marrow diseases (aplastic anemia, myelodisplastic syndromes)
Severe sepsis
Autoimmune disease like lupus erythematosis

The above information applies to the total white blood cell count, but as mentioned above there are five different types of white blood cells that will be included in your complete blood count. These five cell types are neutrophils, eosinophils, basophils, lymphocytes and monocytes. They will be discussed individually.

Neutrophils

Constitute sixty to seventy percent of all white blood cells. These are the cells that combat bacteria. Once your body is invaded by bacteria, neutrophils, utilizing an impressive array of chemicals, kill the invader in a process known as phagocytosis. Neutrophils will increase in response to bacterial infection, inflammatory disease, chronic myelogenous leukemia, or other bone marrow disorders. They will decrease in response to very severe bacterial infection (bone marrow exhaustion) and certain medications.

Eosinophils

Constitute two to four percent of all white blood cells. Eosinophils are brought to the fray by allergies. They combat the effect of histamine, the cause of allergic reactions. They react to inflammation of the skin and they will kill some parasitic invaders. Some infections and bone marrow disorders will activate them as well. They will be reduced in severe infections when neutrophils are called to fight.

Basophils

Constitute one half to one percent of all white blood cells. They intensify the allergic response by liberating heparin, histamine and serotonin in allergic reactions. They can be increased in leukemia, hypersensitivity reaction to food and chronic inflammation.

Lymphocytes

Total lymphocytes constitute twenty-five percent of all white blood cells. This cell is important in mediating immune responses. There are three principle types of lymphocytes: B cells that turn into plasma cells that manufacture antibodies, a protein that is formed in response to a specific invader; T cells that attack viruses, cancer cells and transplanted organs; natural killer T cells that kill bacteria and cancer cells. An elevation of total lymphocytes is caused by the acute phase of many viral illnesses, chronic infections like tuberculosis, lymphatic malignancies including chronic lymphocytic leukemia, overactive thyroid gland, Addison's disease and connective tissue diseases. Lymphocytes are reduced in AIDS, any disease that destroys the bone marrow such as cancer or aplastic anemia, use of steroids, multiple sclerosis, myasthenia gravis and Guillain Barre syndrome (autoimmune inflammation of nerve cells often occurring five days to three weeks after an infection, surgery, or vaccination).

Monocytes

Three to eight percent of all white blood cells. These cells transform into a cell known as a macrophage. Macrophages either wander about the body or become fixed in different organs such as the liver, brain and lung. Their responsibility is phagocytosis (they kill and digest unwanted invaders). An increased monocyte count can occur in chronic inflammatory disease, tuberculosis, multiple myeloma, parasitic infections and some viral infections like infectious mononucleosis, measles and mumps. Monocytes are decreased in aplastic anemia and cortisone use.

2. Red blood cells. The purpose of your red blood cells is to carry oxygen from the lungs to the rest of your body. In addition, the red blood cells pick up carbon dioxide (a waste product from your cells). The carbon dioxide is then released into your lungs where it is exhaled.

A low red blood cell count indicates anemia, of which there are many varieties. A high red blood count indicates polycythemia vera. In this condition the blood is 'too thick,' and this creates a risk of clumping, which could lead to blockage of small blood vessels leading to a wide variety of symptoms depending on the blood vessel involved.

Hematocrit. This test is a measure of the volume of blood caused by the red blood cells as compared to the liquid portion of the blood (plasma). For instance, a hematocrit of forty-two percent means that the red blood cells occupy forty-two percent of the total blood volume and the plasma occupies the remainder, except for a small amount occupied by white blood cells.

Hemoglobin. This is a complex molecule containing iron. Hemoglobin is located in the red blood cells. It serves as the carrier of oxygen and is responsible for the blood's red color. The measure of hemoglobin is a good indicator of the ability of the red blood cells to carry oxygen throughout the body.

Red blood cell indices. There are three red blood cell indices. They are the mean corpuscular volume (MCV), mean corpuscular hemoglobin (MCH), and mean corpuscular hemoglobin concentration (MCHC).

The MCV shows the size of the red blood cells. The MCH value is the amount of hemoglobin in an average red blood cell. The MCHC measures the concentration of hemoglobin in an average red blood cell. These numbers are important to differentiate between the various types of anemia. The red cell distribution width (RDW) measures the different sizes of red blood cells that are present.

ELEVATION (Red blood cells)

Polycythemia vera
Kidney disease
Chronic lung disease (pulmonary fibrosis)
Right sided heart failure
Severe dehydration
Medication (anabolic steroid)
Smoking
Living at a high altitude (physiological response)

REDUCTION

Acute bleeding
Chronic bleeding
Many medications including chemotherapy drugs
Chronic diseases (kidney failure, malignancies, inflammatory bowel diseases)
Iron deficiency
Vitamin deficiency
Endocrine gland underactivity (hypothyroidism)
Autoimmune diseases (lupus)

3. Platelet count. Platelets are the smallest type of blood cell (actually not a full cell with a nucleus like all your other cells, but rather a fragment of a cell). They are important in the clotting of the blood. If you bleed for whatever reason, the platelets clump together and form a plug that helps to stop the bleeding. The normal platelet count is 150,000 to 450,000.

If there are too many platelets (thrombocytosis) you are at risk of a blood clot spontaneously forming in a blood vessel. If there are too few platelets (thrombocytopenia) there is a risk of spontaneous uncontrolled bleeding.

ELEVATION

Unknown cause
Infection
Post surgery
Polycythemia vera
Chronic myelogenous leukemia
Genetic mutation

REDUCTION

Leukemia or other bone marrow disorder
Medication
Autoimmune disorder (idiopathic thrombocytopenic purpura)

Blood smear: In this test a drop of blood is smeared on a slide and then stained with a special dye. The slide is then examined under a microscope and the various blood cells, red and white, are described and counted. This provides clues to the type of blood disorder you may have.

Needless to say a blood count can provide valuable clues concerning your state of health. It is a vital part of the screening process: it can detect anemia or polycythemia; it can provide valuable clues to uncover the reason for weakness, weight loss, elevated temperature, easy bruising and infection; it can diagnose leukemia; it can follow the course of chemotherapy or radiation or certain drug effects; it can determine the reason for abnormal bleeding.

COMPLETE URINALYSIS

1. An evaluation of the color.

Normally the color varies from colorless to dark yellow. Much depends upon the amount of liquid consumed and the type of food ingested. Beets may turn the urine red. Blood in the urine may be visible as red if it is in large volume or tea color if it is in smaller volume. Blood in the urine can also only be seen microscopically, so the absence of the red or tea color may not mean that there is no blood. Jaundice will turn urine the color of strong tea. Some medications can also turn urine different colors.

2. The specific gravity measures the concentration of the urine.

The specific gravity of water is 1.000. The normal specific gravity of urine is 1.006 to 1.030 (somewhat 'thicker' than water). The specific gravity depends upon the amount of liquid and solid food ingested. A constant low specific gravity suggests kidney damage, indicating that the kidney has lost the ability to concentrate the urine.

3. The urine ph is a measure of the alkalinity or acidity of the urine.

It depends on what we eat. A neutral ph is 7.0. An acidic ph is less than 7, and an alkaline ph is more than 7. Our kidneys manage to keep our urine ph between 6 and 7.4, but it may range from 4.5 to 8.

An increase in the acidity of the urine occurs with uncontrolled diabetes mellitus, dehydration, starvation, diarrhea, and lung diseases where breathing is hampered resulting in less ability of the lungs to eliminate your bodies carbon dioxide cellular waste product.

An increase in the alkalinity of the urine occurs with some kidney diseases, aspirin poisoning and lung diseases involving increased respiratory rates where the carbon dioxide is more rapidly exhaled.

The ph of the urine tends to acidity, but vegetarians produce more alkaline urine. If your urine is more alkaline and it persists, it could be possible that you

have a urinary tract infection. Most of the bacteria that cause an infection make
the urine alkaline.

Some types of kidney stones form in acidic urine. In these cases an attempt is
made to keep the urine alkaline. Other types of stones form in alkaline urine. In
this case the urine should be kept acidic.

4. Urine sugar

If your blood sugar is too high (as seen in diabetes mellitus), when the blood
passes through the kidney to be filtered some of the excess sugar will spill over
into the urine. Normally there is no sugar in the urine, so the presence of same is
indicative of diabetes mellitus—unless you have a condition (rare) known as renal
glycosuria where even with normal blood sugar there is still a spillage of the blood
sugar into the urine. There have been patients wrongly diagnosed with diabetes
who have had renal glycosuria. Also a number of medications have caused false
positive results for urine sugar.

On the strength of an elevated urine sugar test a patient was given diabetic
medication. The only problem was that the patient had renal glycosuria, and the
diabetic medication resulted in hypoglycemis (low blood sugar) severe enough to
cause her to have a seizure. The moral of the story is that if you test positive for
urine sugar, the diagnosis of diabetes mellitus or renal glycosuria should be confirmed by a blood sugar test.

5. Protein

Protein in the urine always means kidney disease. The amount of protein (albumin) correlates directly with the severity of the kidney disease.

6. Bilirubin

If bilirubin is elevated in the urine, this is a sign of liver disease or disease of the
bile ducts or suggests increased breakdown of red blood cells (hemolysis).

7. Urobilinogin

Small traces of urobilinogen are normal in the urine. Bacteria, normally in your
intestine, form urobilinogen from bilirubin. Some of the urobilinogen is reabsorbed into the circulation by liver cells and then is excreted into the urine by the
kidneys. If there are large amounts of bilirubin being formed, such as in liver disease or hemolysis, then excessive amounts of urobilinogen may appear in the
urine. Of interest is that the urobilinogen remaining in the intestine that has not

been reabsorbed is chemically converted to another substance called stercobilin, which gives feces their characteristic brown color. In bile duct obstruction very little bilirubin reaches the intestine, so little is converted to urobilinogen and the feces may become very light in color.

8. Nitrites and leucocyte esterase

Leucocyte esterase is an enzyme that is released by white blood cells. Most urinary tract bacteria cause nitrates from your diet to be converted to nitrites. Neither nitrites nor leucocyte esterase is normally present in the urine, so either one or both of these tests, if positive in the urine, indicate an infection by certain varieties of bacteria.

9. Microscopic examination of the urine:

The fresh urine is centrifuged and the sediment is collected from the bottom of the centrifuge tube and placed upon a glass slide for microscopic examination. White blood cells and red blood cells are then counted. The normal range for white blood cells is zero to five per high powered microscopic field. More than this number could mean infection and a urine culture may need to be done. There should be no more than three red blood cells per high powered field in the urine. If there are more, the cause of the urinary bleeding should be determined. The possibilities are: stone, bacterial infection, trauma, tumor, tuberculosis or fungal infection.

The microscopic urinalysis may also demonstrate casts, which are coagulated protein (albuminous) material that form in the kidney tubules under abnormal conditions. They are rounded and cylindrical. Casts in the urine are a sure sign of a kidney disorder. Six types of kidney casts have been identified as follows:

Hyaline casts are colorless and transparent. They are the most frequent type identified, and indicate early kidney disease.

Granular casts (casts with granules in them) indicate severe kidney disease. They may also appear following strenuous exercise, so this aspect of the history must be known.

Waxy casts are degenerated granular casts. They are seen in severe kidney disease causing chronic kidney failure which may be due to malignant hypertension or diabetes mellitus.

Red cell casts indicate a severe degree of kidney bleeding.

White cell casts indicate severe infection.

Fatty casts contain fat droplets. They can be seen in a number of medical conditions and when kidneys are poisoned by toxic substances such as heavy metals.

BLOOD CHEMICAL PROFILE

Refers to a group of blood tests that together give you important information about your state of health.

The tests include:

Glucose (sugar)

The normal blood glucose is: fasting—70 to 99; Two hours after a meal—70 to 145; random test—70 to 125. Carbohydrates are ingested and turned into glucose by the body. Glucose provides the energy for your body cells. Insulin (manufactured by your pancreas) accelerates the transport of glucose into body cells where it is used for energy.

ELEVATION

Diabetes mellitus
Heart attack and stroke (transient elevation)
Cushing's syndrome
Acromegaly

REDUCTION

Diabetic medication (oral diabetic medication and insulin injections)
Fasting
Underactive adrenal gland, thyroid gland, pituitary gland
Cancer
Infections
Pancreatic tumor (insulinoma)
Adrenal tumor (pheochromocytoma)
Liver disease

Blood Urea Nitrogen (BUN)

Urea is formed due to the breakdown of protein in your body. A normal functioning kidney will then excrete the urea.

ELEVATION

Kidney failure
Heart failure
Shock
Dehydration
Upper gastrointestinal bleeding
High protein diets
Some medications
Burns

REDUCTION

Some liver disease
Decreased protein intake
Excessive water intake or intravenous fluids (dilution effect)
Some liver diseases

Creatinine

Creatine is a compound that all your muscles use to produce energy in order to contract. When creatine is broken down it forms a waste product known as creatinine. The kidney's job is to excrete this creatinine in the urine, therefore the blood level of creatinine is a good measure of your kidney function. When elevated in the blood it suggests the kidney's function is reduced. Since the amount of creatinine produced depends upon your size and muscle mass, a man will have a slightly higher creatinine than a woman or child.

ELEVATION

Kidney failure
Dehydration
Muscular dystrophy (early stage)
Heart failure

REDUCTION

Muscular dystrophy (late stage)
Myasthenis Gravis
Pregnancy

Uric acid

Foods and nucleic acids (DNA) are broken down in your body. The result of that breakdown is uric acid, another waste product that the body has to get rid of. Two thirds is excreted by your kidneys and one third is excreted in your feces. Low uric acid levels cause no problems, but high uric acid levels cause a condition known as gout. This condition is either caused when uric acid is overproduced, or your kidneys fail to excrete it. High uric acid levels can deposit in your joints causing a crippling, painful and deforming arthritis.

ELEVATION

Gout
Kidney failure
High purine diets
Obesity
Medication (aspirin, diuretics, antihypertensives, chemotherapy)
Radiation
Malignancies (leukemia, lymphoma)

REDUCTION

Usually not clinically significant, but can be reduced in:
Wilson's disease
Fanconi syndrome
Obstructive biliary disease

Electrolytes

Included in this category are four tests: sodium, chloride, potassium, bicarbonate. When you measure bicarbonate, you are actually measuring the amount of carbon dioxide in your body, an end product of your cell's metabolism, which is eventually eliminated from the body through your lungs. All these minerals are responsible for keeping body fluids in balance, and are critical for the proper functioning of your muscles, heart and other organs.

Sodium
ELEVATION

Primary aldosteronism
Cushing's syndrome
Diabetes insipidus
Kidney failure
Water deprivation
High salt diet

REDUCTION

Congestive heart failure
Kidney disease
Hypothyroidism
Syndrome of innapropriate secretion of antidiuretic hormone
Brain hemorrhage, tumor, trauma, or abscess
Addison's disease
Hypopituitarism
Acute intermittent porphyrias
Cirrhosis
Increased sweating
Burns

Chloride

Follows sodium as sodium chloride (salt)

Potassium

Most of the potassium in your body is in your cells, therefore the amount in your red blood cells is much greater than the amount in your plasma (the liquid part of the blood). After your blood is drawn, and if the test tube is inadvertently shaken up injuring red blood cells, these cells may leak potassium in the sample which will falsely elevate potassium.

Kidneys control the amount of potassium excreted in the urine. That is why kidney failure causes an elevated potassium, which can have adverse effects on your heart. So too can a reduced potassium.

ELEVATION

Kidney failure
Addison's disease
Excessive potassium ingestion
Destruction of red blood cells due to burns or injury
Medication (angiotensin converting enzyme inhibitors—used for blood pressure control)

REDUCTION

Reduced kidney function
Diuretics
Primary aldosteronism
Severe vomiting or diarrhea
Eating disorders including excessive use of laxatives

Bicarbonate

Bicarbonate prevents the body tissues from becoming too acidic. Kidneys and lungs balance the level of bicarbonate in the body, so if the bicarbonate is too high or low it suggests a malfunction of either or both of those organs.

ELEVATION

Primary aldosteronism
Cushing's syndrome
Respiratory illnesses (breathing disorders)
Severe vomiting

REDUCTION

Diabetic ketoacdosis or lactic acidosis
Diarrhea
Kidney disease
Aspirin overdose
Methanol or ethylene glycol poisoning
Addison's disease

Calcium

Calcium comes from the food you eat. It is absorbed into the blood stream and is stored in your teeth and bones. In the blood, most of the calcium is bound to protein (albumin), but a small percent of it circulates in a free form and plays a vital role in cardiac function, blood clotting, release of hormones, muscle contractions and nerve transmission. It is controlled by a hormone of the parathyroid gland called parathormone and is also controlled by vitamin D, a fat soluble vitamin that is found in food and also can be made in your skin by sunlight. Once made, the vitamin D promotes the absorption of calcium from food in your gastrointestinal tract.

ELEVATION

Hyperparathyroidism
Excessive ingestion of calcium or vitamin D
Medications (lithium, thiazide diuretics)
Cancer (breast, lung, blood)
Sarcoidosis
Addison's disease
Kidney dialysis
Hyperthyroidism
Familial hypocalciuric hypercalcemia (a genetic disorder)
Paget's disease
Milk alkali syndrome

REDUCTION

Hypoparathyroidism
Vitamin D deficiency
Malnutrition and low albumin levels
Malabsorption
Common medications including anticonvulsants and barbiturates
Kidney failure
Pancreatitis

Phosphorus

Phosphorus is a component of many proteins and nucleic acid in our DNA. It is necessary for normal bone and tooth structure. An elevated phosphorus blood level almost always indicates abnormal kidney function. On occasion the cause may be due to excessive intake of phosphorus or vitamin D, which, like calcium, increases the absorption of phosphorus from the intestines. Most of your phosphorus is stored in your cells, so it may be elevated in your blood during hemolysis of red blood cells and breakdown of muscle cells.

ELEVATION

Kidney failure
Low calcium levels
Hypoparathyroidism
Increased dietary intake of phosphates
Bone metatstases
Liver disease
Sarcoidosis

REDUCTION

Hyperparathyroidism
Elevated calcium
Inadequate dietary intake of phosphates
Diabetic ketoacidosis
Hyperinsulinism

Bilirubin

As previously mentioned, when red blood cells have lived out their three month life-span they are broken down. One of the breakdown products is bilirubin. It is picked up by the liver and is secreted into the gall bladder as bile and stored. When stimulated by eating, the gall bladder contracts and sends bilirubin into the bile duct and then into the small intestine to help digest fat.

ELEVATION

Hemolysis (increased breakdown of red blood cells)
Hepatitis
Liver failure
Gilbert's syndrome
Medications
Bile duct obstruction (due to stone or tumor)

REDUCTION

Not clinically significant

SGOT (AST)

Serum glutamic oxalacetic transaminase is an enzyme produced in the liver and the heart. It is also called AST aspartate aminotransferase. When the liver or heart are damaged (hepatitis—heart attack) the enzyme leaks out and the level in the blood becomes elevated.

ELEVATION

Heart Attack
Liver disease
Pancreatitis
Muscular dystrophy
Stroke
Alcoholism
Congestive heart failure
Testicular or ovarian hypofunction

REDUCTION

Vitamin B6 deficiency

SGPT (ALT)

Serum glutamic pyruvate transaminase is an enzyme also produced in the liver and heart. It is also called alanine aminotransferase (ALT). If SGOT is elevated, SGPT will follow, but to a lesser extent.

LDH

Lactic dehydrogenase is an enzyme found in the brain, heart muscle, skeletal muscle, kidneys, lungs and blood cells. There are five forms of this enzyme each located in higher concentration in specific tissues. The total LDH is performed on the screening test. If the total LDH is elevated, it tells you that something is wrong and further evaluation should be made.

ELEVATION

Heart attack

Stroke
Liver disease
Pancreatitis
Muscle disease
Pulmonary Embolus (blood clot)
Intestinal injury
Hemolysis
Infectious mononucleosis
Pernicious anemia
Drugs
Kidney disease
Some cancers

REDUCTION

Not clinically significant

Alkaline phosphatase (ALP)

An enzyme found in the liver, blood, intestines and bone cells. The chemical structure of this enzyme varies depending on where it has been produced (liver or bone). Testing allows your physician to determine the origin of the elevation. When children's bones grow, the alkaline phosphatase will be normally very high, but an elevated alkaline phosphatase in an adult is abnormal and demands a search for the cause. Alkaline phosphatase levels in children decrease to normal adult levels between the ages of sixteen and twenty. During the third trimester of pregnancy, the levels may be twice the normal adult range, and they return to normal about a month after delivery

ELEVATION

Liver:
Liver disease of any kind including cancer
Medications

Bone:
Paget's disease
Cancer (all types and multiple myeloma)
Fracture
Osteomalacia

Rickets

Others conditions causing alkaline phosphatase elevations:
ELEVATION

Hypothyroidism
Kidney disease (secondary hyperparathyroidism)
Polycythemia Vera
Myelofibrosis
Bile duct obstruction
Oral contraceptives
Pregnancy

REDUCTION

Chronic myelogenous leukemia
Pernicious anemia
Aplastic anemia
Malnutrition

Total protein

Proteins are important parts of all body cells and tissues. Some examples of proteins we have already discussed are: enzymes, hormones, antibodies (immunoglobulins) and hemoglobin. Blood proteins are divided into two groups—albumin and globulins. The total protein is the sum of albumin and globulins in your body.

ELEVATION

Chronic infection
Multiple myeloma
Waldenstrom's disease

REDUCTION

Hemorrhage
Extensive burns
Liver disease
Malabdorption
Malnutrition
Glomerulonephritis

Protein losing enteropathy
Light chain disease

LDL Cholesterol

Cholesterol is a lipid (fatty) substance used to form cell membranes and some hormones. Fatty substances like cholesterol cannot dissolve in the blood stream, so they are carried in the blood combined with protein called lipoproteins. There are two types of lipoproteins: low density lipoproteins (LDL) and high-density lipoproteins (HDL).

LDL is the principle carrier of cholesterol in the blood. If the concentration of LDL is too high, it can cause blocked arteries and result in heart attack or stroke. This is the reason LDL is called "bad cholesterol." You acquire cholesterol in two ways: ingesting it and by your liver producing it. Your liver produces all the cholesterol you need, so theoretically you needn't consume it. Foods from animals contain cholesterol. Food from fruits and vegetables do not contain cholesterol. Your total cholesterol intake should be limited. Saturated fats and trans fats cause plaque build up in arteries and should be avoided.

HOW TO LOWER AN ELEVATED LDL CHOLSTEROL

1. Low-saturated fat, low cholesterol eating plan that avoids weight gain. The plan should not have more than seven percent of calories from saturated fat and should have less than 200 milligrams of cholesterol per day.

2. Weight management: Lose weight if you are overweight.

3. Exercise at least thirty minutes every day. Especially important for those with an elevated triglyceride and a large waist measurement (more than 40 inches in men and 35 inches in women).

4. Eat at least two servings of soluble fiber per day (oats, fruits, vegetables, legumes).

5. Medication, principally the statin family of drugs.

HDL cholesterol

HDL cholesterol constitutes about thirty percent of the blood cholesterol. HDL cholesterol removes excess cholesterol from artery blockages (plaques) and thus slows down their growth. It is for this reason that HDL is called "good cholesterol", so the higher the better. Exercise raises HDL cholesterol. If you smoke—stop. If you're overweight—try to lose the excess.

HOW TO INCREASE A LOW HDL CHOLESTEROL

1. Exercise at least four days per week and try to elevate your heart rate for twenty to thirty minutes at a time.

2. Lose weight.

3. Stop smoking.

4. Stop trans fats.

5. Discontinue more than one or two drinks of alcohol per day.

6. Eat at least two servings per day of soluble fiber.

7. Eat monounsaturated fats (peanut butter, avacado oil, canola oil)

8. Omega 3 fatty acids

9. Niacin

10. Medication

Triglyceride

The largest percentage of fat in the diet and in your fatty tissue is in the form of triglycerides. Elevated triglycerides have been correlated with a higher risk for heart attack and stroke. This is especially true if you have other risk factors such as obesity or diabetes.

HOW TO DECREASE AN ELEVATED TRIGLYCERIDE

Lose weight
Discontinue alcohol
Reduce trans fats, saturated fat and cholesterol in your diet
Exercise
Reduce carbohydrate
Take Omega 3 fatty acids (fish or capsules)
Control diabetes

This concludes the discussion of the screening laboratory data. Once these results are available, your physician will add this information to his already growing data base from the history and physical examination. In most instances he will have a firm diagnosis. In some instances further testing will be necessary.

PART IV
SUMMARY

◆

Take charge of your health
Summary list

You have finished the three parts of your complete medical examination.

During the history, you and your physician have gotten to know each other. Hopefully you have met a compassionate person that has demonstrated expertise and performed a complete and thorough physical examination. Without these, your relationship may be off to a bad start. Was your physician a good listener? Was he patient? Was he caring? Was his examination thorough? Did he answer all your questions? Your future relationship, and even your response to his suggestions, may rest upon the answer to these questions.

Now that you have completed the three step process one of three things will happen:

1. Your physician may report that he can't find a thing wrong with you. Your history was unrevealing, your physical examination was entirely normal and your screening laboratory data all fell within normal limits. At this point you will receive whatever advice he may offer and happily leave and return for another exam when your physician suggests it may be necessary. The timing will depend upon your age and perhaps your family history.

2. Your physician will have enough information to tell you exactly what your diagnosis is and what you must do in terms of therapy and future follow up evaluations.

3. Or he will have developed a list of possible diagnosis that must now be further investigated in order to pin point a single diagnosis or multiple diagnoses. This will require further diagnostic testing. He may order x-rays, MRI or CT scan, further blood studies or urine samples etc.

4. He may refer you to another physician because he has uncovered a problem outside of his area of expertise, and best left in more experienced hands.

Once the process related to the above four possibilities has been completed, you are now in a position to be a take charge patient. At this point you have had all your questions answered, and you should have a full understanding about all your diagnoses and therapy. This is the key to taking a leadership role. You and your physician need to decide when follow up examinations are necessary. If any new diagnosis develops it must be add to your diagnostic list and determined how it impacts your current diagnoses.

CLINICAL EXAMPLE

I am reminded of a patient who was about to undergo elective surgery. This lady had a list of questions for her anesthesiologist. I know her well, and she is the type of person who receives comfort based upon full disclosure and knowledge of what she is about to face, good or bad. She and Google are on intimate terms. She met her anesthesiologist for the first time the morning of surgery. He introduced himself, took a brief history, listened to her heart and lungs and reviewed her chart. When he completed this quick introduction, the patient told him that she had a list of questions for him. "How many?" he said. The patient held up a sheet of paper with about ten written questions. "About ten," was the reply. "I'll answer three," he said with an impatient look on his face. The shattered patient got her three questions rapidly answered, but then went into surgery depressed and scared. Such pre-operative preparation is not conducive to good outcomes (as has been proven many times), and sure enough this patient had a stormy postoperative course. Later she confided in me and told me the whole story. "It made me angry at the whole medical profession," she said. I suggested to her that at that time she should have taken charge of her health. She should have told the anesthesiologist to take the time (probably no more than five minutes) to answer the questions that were important to her. If he still refused, then she should have told the anesthesiologist that he needed to get in touch with her surgeon (the captain of her surgical team) immediately, because unless she had the questions answered, she was prepared to refuse to have the surgery performed at this time and in this place, and she would tell the surgeon the reason for her decision and request another anesthesiologist. Unfortunately, most patients are too meek to assert themselves in this manner, but who has more right?!

Having now undergone this thorough and complete physical examination, you are armed with knowledge about yourself, and research has demonstrated that if you get actively involved in your care you will get better results. Your physicians should welcome your efforts on your own behalf. Not only will you be better prepared emotionally, but your physician will know that you are sure of your decision, and you both understand that the decision has been made together. Two minds are usually better than one. A confident patient is a patient who will have a better outcome.

Once your examination has been completed, and possibly with the help of a few follow up visits, your physician will be in a position to record your final problems in the medical record. This is called a summary list and it includes:

1. Established significant medical diagnosis of a chronic nature that must be followed long term and is vital to current and future decision making. For example, diabetes mellitus, congestive heart failure, hypertension, Crohn's disease, osteoarthritis, multiple sclerosis, manic depressive disorder.

2. Allergies to drugs, and the type of allergic reaction.

3. Known significant surgical or invasive procedures that have been performed. For example, quadruple coronary artery bypass graft, hip replacement, cholecystectomy (gall bladder removal), total abdominal hysterectomy (removal of uterus, fallopian tubes, ovaries), breast biopsy, appendectomy. Listing an old appendectomy is important if, in the future, your physician will have to make a diagnosis as to the cause of lower abdominal pain.

4. Important symptoms should be listed by your doctor if he has not yet established a reason for the symptom. Once the symptom is explained, the diagnosis can displace the symptom. For example: left arm pain subsequently discovered to be due to coronary artery disease.

5. A social risk factor that may be impacting your health. For example: a bitter divorce.

6. Medication list (name and dose) including complementary medications (herbs), vitamins, prescription medications and over the counter medications taken on a regular basis.

7. Immunizations

An example of a medical summary list:

1. Status post quadruple artery bypass graft (anterior descending branch, right, two diagonal branches) 1966

2. Post cardiotomy syndrome—resolved

3. Anemia secondary to cardura and hytrin (resolved when medications discontinued)

4. Elevated total cholesterol and reduced HDL cholesterol (resolved with therapy)

5. Premature atrial contractions

6. Hypertension

7. Benign prostatic hypertrophy

8. Right inguinal herniorrhaphy 1998

9. Cataract surgery (right) 2005 (left) 2007

Medication:

Toprol 100 mgm—one every morning

Hydrochlorothiazide 25 mgm—one every morning

Saw palmetto 320 mgm—one every morning

Centrum Silver multivitamin—one every morning

Omega 3 fatty acids 1000 mgm—one every morning and evening

Flo max 0.4 mgm—two every evening

Lisinopril 20 mgm—two every evening

Simvastatin 10 mgm—one every evening

Halfprim (aspirin) 162 mgm—one every evening

Another example of a medical summary list:

1. Atrial fibrillation

2. Hypertension

3. Degenerative arthritis both knees

4. Endometrial hyperplasia (resolved—see problem 5)

5. Total abdominal hysterectomy 1994

Medication:

Norvasc 5 mgm every morning

Furosemide 20 mgm every morning

Atacand 32 mgm every morning

Ziac 5/6.25 every morning

Warfarin Sodium 4mgm every evening except 2 mgm Tue and Thur

The above examples represent a snapshot of your medical history. It serves as a reminder for you and your personal physician plus others who may be involved in your care.

The medical record is yours, and you are entitled to ask for copies. At a minimum, I would suggest that you ask for the laboratory and any imaging data and the summary list. Keep this record in a permanent file and update it as your conditions or medications change, new diagnoses are established, new allergies develop, or procedures are performed. Keep this list on your person at all times, or place it in a computer file or drawer at home where you and your family will have easy access to it. This record can be enormously helpful—maybe life saving—should you have an unexpected interaction with a new physician.

You have taken the first step in controlling your health and preventing medical errors. By learning all about your state of health, you are prepared to take your place as the leading member of your health care team. You have learned about your diagnoses from your physician. In this day and age, you have further resources to educate you. Principle among these sources is the internet. Type in a few words, click, and the total information on any subject is there at your fingertips. You will learn much as you surf the net, and it may bring many more questions to your mind. Your physician should answer these questions for you. This communication is best done in person as opposed to phone calls, but either way, satisfy your self that you have received the answer. If you don't understand, you must ask again. You need a clear, informed mind to assist you in making what often are critically important decisions. You will need to put your trust in a doctor you can trust. He is in the best position to lead you through what is often a maze of possibilities, options and opinions.

In summary:

Be sure that you avail yourself of a COMPLETE MEDICAL EXAMINATION.
You now know what it entails.

When the examination is complete and you have all the results in the form of
a summary list, keep it on your person or anyplace where you would have instant
access.

As any part of the summary list changes, update the list to keep it current.

If you do the above you will be in a good position to inform your physicians
or any new healthcare professionals you may come in contact with. This could be
crucial to prevent medical errors. TAKE CHARGE OF YOUR HEALTH.

PART V

THE PREVENTION OF MEDICAL ERRORS

✦

"ES IRRT DER MENSCH, SO LANG ER STREBT"

Johann Wolfgang von Goethe
(1749–1832)

Ninety-eight thousand people per year die as a result of medical errors, a number that represents more deaths than occur from automobile accidents or breast cancer. This statistic was published by the Institute of Medicine in 1999, and has prompted efforts by the Joint Commission on Accreditation of Healthcare Organizations to focus the accreditation process on operational systems critical to the safety and quality of patient care.

My first inclination on reading this statistic was disbelief. What is the Institute of Medicine? Are they a governmental organization? How are they funded?

The federal government created the National Academy of Sciences to serve as an advisor on scientific matters. However, the Academy and its associated organization (e.g. the Institute of Medicine) is a private, non-governmental organization that does not receive direct federal appropriations for their work. The Institute of Medicine's charter establishes it as an independent body. They use unpaid volunteer experts who author their reports. Each report undergoes a rigorous and formal peer review process that must be evidence-based where possible, or noted as an expert opinion where not possible. Many meetings of the Institute of Medicine are open to the public, but the committee may deliberate amongst themselves. They must reach consensus, and any potential conflict of interest could disqualify a committee member.

So, far be it from me to dispute this committee's findings—and the Joint Commission must have taken it seriously as well, for they have launched their nationwide effort to minimize medical errors in healthcare organizations.

Now that we have accepted the fact that medical errors occur, let's define what medical errors are. There is a long list of hospital errors that have resulted in death or injury, and they are recorded and categorized by the Joint Commission as so-called sentinel events. This is necessary so that the Joint Commission can investigate and make sure that the hospital has put systems in place to prevent the error from reoccurring. These sentinel events are:

• Anesthesia related: death or injury resulting from anesthesia.

- Delay in treatment: Treatment delays may result from failure to diagnose in a timely manner, or incorrectly diagnose. Both of these may result in disability or death. This is the reason the complete medical examination is so crucial.

- Elopement: when a patient leaves a facility of his own accord before diagnosis and/or treatment have been started or completed.

- Infection-related: Lapses in sterile technique may result in an infection causing disability or death.

- Maternal Deaths: Deaths occurring during obstetrical delivery.

- Medical Equipment: Medical equipment failures may result in disability or death.

- Medication error: Physician, pharmacist, or patient error may result in injury or death due to improper or wrong medication use.

- Operative/Post-operative: Complications resulting from surgical or post surgical care.

- Patient Abduction: The abduction of a newborn infant from the newborn nursery.

- Patient Falls: The failure to identify the fall-risk patient, and/or the failure to safeguard the patient may result in severe injury or death.

- Perinatal Deaths/Injury: injuries or death occurring around the time of birth.

- Potassium Chloride: The accidental direct intravenous injection of potassium chloride can result in cardiac arrest.

- Restraint Deaths: Restraints must be used only as a last resort to protect patients from themselves and staff from the patient. Restraints must be used only for the shortest time necessary and restrained patients must be monitored on a regular basis. Failure to properly monitor these patients may result in medical complications or death.

- Suicide: Guidelines must be in place to identify and monitor the suicidal patient. Failure to adhere to these guidelines may result in injury or death.

- Transfusion: An improperly matched blood transfusion could result in severe injury or death.

- Ventilator: Mechanical ventilation using ventilators is often necessary to breathe for patients who are unable to breathe for themselves. Improper ventilator settings, machine failure and incomplete monitoring may result in death.

- Wrong site surgery: Failure to identify the precise surgical site may lead to wrong-site surgery.

Medical errors do not only happen within hospitals. They can occur anywhere healthcare is delivered, including outpatient surgery centers, clinics, doctors' offices, nursing homes, pharmacies and patient's homes. In fact, home care fires are another sentinel event. Patients over sixty-five have fallen victim to home care fires. Risk factors identified are: 1) living alone, 2) absence of a working smoke detector, 3) flammable clothing, 4) home oxygen, 5) cognitive impairment, 6) smoking. The latter has been a factor in all cases reported.

Errors can occur as the result of incomplete medical history taking and failure to perform a careful physical examination. I deem these two factors as critically important, and thus again my emphasis on the value of a properly performed complete history and physical examination.

Clearly, when a medical error has occurred there has been a breakdown of one or more of the built-in safety measures put in place to prevent such mishaps. These safety measures are the responsibility of your healthcare team, but as mentioned above—do not leave it to them alone! You must get involved. Take some responsibility for your care. Don't sit by as a passive member of the team. You are the most important member, so ask questions! Satisfy yourself that what you are about to do is the best option that can be taken now for you to receive an optimal result.

As mentioned, the Joint Commission has recommended patient safety standards for all healthcare organizations. These standards are updated and published every year. It is then the organization's responsibility to see to it that these safety standards are implemented in a manner suiting their organization's culture.

The safety standards are developed for the following healthcare organizations:

1.   Ambulatory Care and Office-Based Surgery

2.   Assisted living

3.   Behavioral Healthcare

4.   Critical Care Hospital and Hospital

5. Disease-Specific Care

6. Home Care

7. Laboratory

8. Long Term Care

9. Networks

These standards are published on the Joint Commission web site: JCAHO.org.

As a patient, you must play a part in assisting these organizations in providing you safe and error-free care.

How can you help?

One of the most common causes of medical errors starts with a written prescription. The mere writing of the prescription is the principle source of the error. If you can't read the prescription easily, then you should assume that the pharmacist will have the same difficulty. Physicians have been made aware of the tragedies that have occurred by poor penmanship, and have been inundated with information about the subject. More and more prescriptions are being typed and uploaded from computers, but the great majority is still hand written. So, if you receive a prescription you can't read, ask that it be rewritten, or at a minimum that it be spelled for you exactly.

If you are hospitalized, and receive a medication that is unfamiliar to you, or appears to have changed, don't take it until the issue has been clarified.

If you are hospitalized, be sure that before anyone gives you your medicine they have checked your identity by looking at your wristband.

If you are to receive a medication at a prescribed time, and it is not forthcoming in a timely manner, be sure that you tell the nurse or physician. The timing of prescribed medications can be crucial to your health.

You should learn the name of your medication, both trade name and generic. Don't rely on your memory alone—keep your summary list available.

Learn about the side effects of the medications you take. If you are experiencing one or more of them, report it to your physician.

If you are taking multiple medications, be sure you are aware of any drug interactions that could occur. For instance, some medications may hinder or enhance blood thinning agents (anticoagulants) and cause serious complications.

Your physician cannot possibly know every drug interaction, so read your pharmacist's instructions or ask him personally. All pharmacists should have drug interaction software computer programs, and they can look it up for you. Your physician also has easy access to these programs.

Always make sure that any physician is aware of all the medications you take. That includes prescription medications, over-the-counter medicines, herbs and vitamins. You should understand what your medication is for, how long it should be taken and what it could interact with, including other medications and food.

If you are hospitalized and receiving intravenous medication, your nurse should know how long the intravenous is supposed to drip before it runs out. If it seems to you that the intravenous fluid is not following that schedule, report it to the nurse.

Whatever raises questions in your mind, or does not seem right—don't keep in your brain unanswered. It will inevitably lead to insecurity and loss of confidence in your physician. So, be sure to ask. Lacking that possibility—look it up. Get the information resolved in your mind. It is too important an issue to remain unanswered.

Always ask about your test results. Do not accept that no news means good news.

Anytime you meet a new member of your healthcare team, be sure that they introduce themselves to you. Check their identification badge. This is a special warning for women with newborns.

Hospital based infections have become a serious problem in healthcare. It has been demonstrated that healthcare workers can carry antibiotic resistant bacteria, viruses and fungi on their hands. Proper hand hygiene can greatly reduce the incidence. Washing with soap and water can be effective if done properly, but it is time consuming, has to be done very often and can result in significant dryness and irritation to the hands. Most hospitals have introduced an alcohol rub hand washing system which can kill bacteria in fifteen seconds, can reduce bacteria count 10,000 fold and is gentle on the hands. If your physician, or another hospital healthcare worker, plans to examine you or treat you, and you notice that he has not washed his hands, insist he do so.

Don't hesitate to ask a physician to explain his experience and specialized training that qualifies him to care for your specific problem. A confident physician will welcome the opportunity.

If you are to undergo an invasive procedure (surgery or test) of any type, you will be asked to sign a consent form. Read it carefully, and if there is anything that you do not understand, ask that it be explained to you. Before you sign the consent form you are entitled to fully understand the nature of the procedure, the benefits that are expected to accrue, other possible alternatives to the procedure and the risks of the procedure.

If after careful evaluation you are still unsure about your diagnosis or treatment options, do not hesitate to seek a second, or even a third opinion. The more information you have about a difficult decision, the more confidence you will have in making it.

If you have had a surgical procedure in a hospital or surgical center, you will receive written and verbal instructions about post-operative care (usually from a nurse). Be sure that you, or an advocate, clearly understand the instructions before you leave. Don't hesitate to clarify your answers, and if you feel the instructions are still vague, and you are still confused, you must speak with your physician for clarification. He will appreciate clarifying the issue for you, rather than you suffering some complication as a result of uncertainty.

Be sure that your surgical site is identified by skin marker. The horror stories about the wrong leg amputation or wrong surgical site operation should never happen.

And lastly, make sure you have a living will and a durable healthcare power of attorney, so that your end-of-life wishes will be respected.

I hope this brief guide has been a help to you. I can't emphasize enough the importance of learning all you can about your health, so you will be in a better position to help guide the course of your diagnosis and treatment.

PART VI
MEDICAL RESOURCES

✦

"Knowledge is of two kinds. We know a subject ourselves, or we know where we can find information upon it."

Samuel Johnson
(1709–1784)

WEB SITES FOR PATIENTS

GOOGLE: Google is not a specific medical web site, but since it has information on anything it can be used as one. A click—and the world's knowledge is at your fingertips. If you are seeking medical information, you can get it on Google. If you are seeking a medical organization and don't know the web site address, type the name of the organization and Google will direct you. I have done this many times.

ALLREFER.COM

Includes extensive information on alternative medicine, diet and nutrition, health news, injuries and wounds, surgery and procedures, symptoms guide, special topics, tests and exams, pictures and images, medical encyclopedia. In addition there are non-medical topics.

CANCER.GOV

This is the web-site for the National Cancer Institute. Every form of cancer is discussed. The most up-to-date information is available and includes: treatment, prevention, genetics, cause, clinical trials, cancer literature, research and related information, screening and testing and statistics.

CENTER FOR DISEASE CONTROL AND PREVENTION (CDC)

Comprehensive information about birth defects, disabilities, diseases and conditions, emergency preparedness and response, environmental health, genetics and genomics, health promotion, injury and violence, travelers health, vaccines and immunizations, workplace safety and health. There are books and journals listed as well as national and state statistics and growth charts.

FAMILYDOCTOR.ORG

Discussion on all conditions from A to Z. Information on healthy living, smart patient guide, women, men, seniors, parents and kids, over the counter guide, health tools. If you are looking for a family physician, type in a zip code, click, and they will be identified.

HEALTHFINDER U.S. DEPARTMENT OF HEALTH AND HUMAN SERVICES

Diseases, conditions and injuries from A to Z, drug database, online checkups, consumer guide, find a provider, find a facility, health news, clinical trials update, weekly health newsletter.

HIV INSITE, UNIVERSITY OF SAN FRANSISCO SCHOOL OF MEDICINE CHI CENTER FOR HIV ONFORMATION

This website provides a comprehensive knowledge base on the latest medical information on HIV, latest research information and preventive measures.

MAYOCLINIC.COM

They have developed a very complete web site that discusses many diseases and conditions. These are written by Mayo Clinic physicians whose picture accompanies the article. They also have information on drugs and supplements, treatment decisions, health living for all ages, health tools including calculators, self assessment tools, quizzes, slide shows, videos and an ask the specialist feature enabling anyone to query one of the Mayo physicians. This web site is my personal favorite that is geared to patients.

MEDLINEPLUS A SERVICE OF THE U.S. NATIONAL LIBRARY OF MEDICINE AND THE NATIONAL INSTITUTE OF HEALTH

Health topics on diseases, conditions and wellness, information on drugs and supplements, medical encyclopedia with pictures and diagrams, medical dictionary, current health news, directory for doctors, dentists and hospitals, local health services, libraries and organizations.

NOAH NEW YORK ONLINE ACCESS TO HEALTH

Disorders and conditions by body locations/systems, local health resources, groups, procedures and medicine, health and wellness, health index from A to Z and page of the month.

WEBMD.COM

They have condition centers with comprehensive information on diseases. There is also information on drugs and herbs, medical library, health tools, find a doctor, clinical trials, health plans and more, women, men, life style, pregnancy and family, diet and nutrition, chats and boards.

BOOKS ON MEDICAL SUBJECTS FOR PATIENTS

JOHNS HOPKIN'S FAMILY HEALTH BOOK

This is an excellent book for patients. It is very comprehensive and includes:

1. Staying healthy: eating well, staying active, staying fit, everyday safety, smoking and how to stop.

2. Healthcare over the life course: family history, genetics and your health, pregnancy and childbirth, infancy, pre-school, teen years, adulthood, senior years.

3. First aid and emergency care

4. Body systems and disorders: an excellent discussion of all body organ systems.

5. Becoming a partner in your healthcare: taking charge of your healthcare, preparing for surgery, how to use medications, home care and long-term care, death and dying.

6. Appendices: medication directory, glossary, growth charts, living wills and advanced directives, measurement conversions, laboratory tests.

7. Color atlas of anatomy, disorders and diseases.

MAYO CLINIC FAMILY HEALTH BOOK

Also an excellent book and it includes:

1. Living well: nutrition, fitness, stress management, other.

2. Common conditions and concerns through life's stages: growth and development, health issues common to children and adults, death and dying.

3. Making sense of your symptoms.

4. First aid and emergency care.

5. Diseases and disorders: signs and symptoms, description of condition, how diagnosed, treatment options.

6. Tests and treatments: tests, medications, surgery, pain management, complementary and alternative therapies.

MERCK MANUAL OF MEDICAL INFORMATION 2ND HOME EDITION

1. Fundamentals.

2. Drugs.

3. Disorders of all organ systems.

THE LIFETIME HEALTH JOURNAL by Karolina Kowiaki

This book will teach you how to keep records of your healthcare throughout your life. This is a critically important issue that will allow you to be able to be an active participant in your healthcare.

1. Introduction.

2. Childhood health record.

3. Adult and long term health record.

NOTHING ABOUT ME WITHOUT ME: A PRACTICAL GUIDE FOR AVOIDING MEDICAL ERRORS by Melinda Ashton M.D. & Linda Richards R.N. MBA

This book is an excellent summary of how to avoid medical errors. There is a patient example illustrating each point.

1. Exploring the issue: aspects of hospital care, patient testing.

2. The many facets of hospital care.

3. Managing medications.

4. Visit to the doctor's office

5. When more than one doctor is involved.

6. Choosing a doctor to satisfy you.

7. When children need medical care.

8. Final thoughts.

HOW TO SAVE YOUR OWN LIFE. THE EIGHT STEPS ONLY YOU CAN TAKE TO MANAGE AND CONTROL YOUR HEALTHCARE by Maria Saved M.D.

1. Trusting yourself as the real expert about your health.

2. Collecting and studying copies of your medical records.

3. Researching your conditions, disease and injuries.

4. Learning which immunizations, exams, and tests you need and when.

5. Helping your doctor help you.

6. Participating in decisions about your treatment options.

7. Knowing how to get the best care in the hospital.

8. Find the courage to treat yourself right.

9. Epilogue: here's to your health.

10. Appendix: copies of actual medical records.

YOU THE SMART PATIENT AN INSIDER'S HANDBOOK TO GETTING THE RIGHT TREATMENT BY Michael F. Roizen M.D. & Mehmet C. Oz M.D.

This book tells readers how to take charge of their own healthcare. The book is written with the collaboration of the Joint Commission, the accrediting organization for all healthcare organizations.

APPENDIX

Computerized Medical History

PAGE 01 MSG-001 07/14/70

    PATIENTS NAME XXXX XXXXXXXX

    DOCTORS NAME SHELDON COHEN

    DATE HISTORY TAKEN 071470

    PATIENT NUMBER XXXXX

    SEX MALE

    AGE 36 YEARS OLD

CHIEF COMPLAINT: TESTS

A. SOCIAL HISTORY:

    1. MARRIED
        NEVER SEPERATED, DIVORCED OR WIDOWED
        CHILDREN: 4
        PRESENTLY MARRIED AND LIVING WITH SPOUSE
        SPOUSE HAS PAYING JOB

    2. OCCUPATION: MASTER MECH

    3. RELIGION: PROTESTANT

    4. CITIZENSHIP: BORN IN U.S.
                  U.S. CITIZEN

    5. EDUCATION: HIGH SCHOOL GRADUATE

    6. MILITARY: SERVED IN ARMED FORCES

      7.   NO TROPICAL COUNTRIES VISITED

      8.   MEDICAL INSURANCE

B. FAMILY HISTORY:

MENTAL OR EMOTIONAL PROBLEMS

CANCER

RHEUMATIC DISEASE

C. GENERAL HEALTH: GOOD

NEVER REFUSED INSURANCE OR MILITARY ENLISTMENT

D. HABITS:

      1.   SMOKED AND INHALED CIGARETTES
           CONTINUING TO DO SO
           ABOUT TWENTY YEARS IN ALL

      2.   ALCOHOLIC BEVERAGES TAKEN
           EXCESSIVELY ABOUT ONCE MONTHLY
           DRINKING PROBLEM DENIED

      3.   NO MEDICATIONS TAKEN REGULARLY

      4.   DENIES EXCESSIVE CONTACT WITH INSECTICIDES, CLEANING FLUID OR OTHER POISONS BY HISTORY

REVIEW OF SYSTEMS: ONLY POSITIVES + PERTINENET NEGATIVES LISTED

      1.   ALLERGY:

WHEEZING

PENICILLIN RECEIVED

PENICILLIN RECEIVED—NO ADVERSE REACTIONS

ASPIRIN RECEIVED

NO ADVERSE REACTION AFTER TAKING ASPIRIN

TETANUS RECEIVED

NO ADVERSE REACTION TO TETANUS SHOT

NO ADVERSE REACTION TO OTHER DRUGS

2. IMMUNIZATIONS:

   SMALLPOX

   TETANUS

   DIPHTHERIA

   POLIO

3. SKIN

   -NO POSITIVE RESPONSES ELICITED

4. ACUTE INFECTIOUS DISEASES

   MEASLES

   WHOOPING COUGH

   MUMPS

   CHICKEN POX

   MD DIAGNOSED ONE OF FOLLOWING:

   SHINGLES, DIPHTHERIA, SCARLET FEVER, TYPHOID FEVER,

   YELLOW FEVER, OR MALARIA

5. OPERATIONS AND INJURIES

   TONSILLECTOMY

6. EYES, EARS, NOSE AND THROAT

   -NO POSITIVE RESPONSES ELICITED

7. RESPIRATORY

   COUGH PRODUCTIVE OF SPUTUM DAILY

   CHEST XRAY WITHIN PAST YEAR—RESULTS UNKNOWN

8. CARDIOVASCULAR:

   CHEST PAIN EXPERIENCED WITHIN LAST YEAR

   BILATERAL

MODERATE IN NATURE

DULL

UNRELATED TO EXERCISE

RELIEVED BY REST

NO RADIATION TO SHOULDER OR ARM

NO NITROGLYCERIN TAKEN

DYSPNEA WITH EXERTION NOTED—INCREASING

ECG WITHIN PAST YEAR

RESULTS UNKNOWN

9. GASTROINTESTINAL:

SUBSTERNAL BURNING—HEART BURN—IN PAST YEAR

SOUR LIQUID COMING UP INTO MOUTH WHEN BENDING OVER

OR LYING DOWN

FREQUENT BELCHING

HEMORRHOIDS

BRIGHT RED BLOOD PASSED WITH BOWEL MOVEMENT

RED BLOOD STREAKED STOOLS NOTED

PAIN WITH BOWEL MOVEMENTS EXPERIENCED

DISCHARGE OR DRAINAGE FROM ANUS OR RECTUM NOTED

10. GENITOURINARY:

-NO POSITIVE RESPONSES ELICITED

11. MALE ENDOCRINE:

-NO POSITIVE RESPONSES ELICITED

12. NEUROLOGICAL:

-NO POSITIVE RESPONSES ELICITED

13. HEMATOLOGY:

    FREQUENT NOSE BLEEDS

    NO BLOOD TRANSFUSIONS

    BRUISES EASILY

14. ENDOCRINE-METABOLISM:

    OVERWEIGHT

    SPECIAL DIET WITHIN PAST YEAR

    WARM WEATHER INTOLERANCE

    EXCESSIVE PERSPIRATION NOTED

15. PSYCHIATRIC:

    ANXIETY

    NO SERIOUS SUICIDAL THOUGHTS

16. JOINTS

    -NO POSITIVE RESPONSES ELICITED

SUBJECTIVE REACTION:

    NO DIFFICULTY WITH QUESTIONS

    LIKE

    FUN

    INTERESTING

***

*** DENOTES POSSIBLE MALFUNCTION PLEASE RECHECK HIS-
TORY AT INDICATED POINTS

END OF HISTORY

You will note that this patient, when asked to type in his chief complaint, instead of describing them on the history, typed in the word 'tests' reflecting his desire to have tests to determine what his problems were. You will further note that there is no heading in this history titled present illness. This computerized medical history was developed with the idea of capturing as much information as possible in all the other categories of the medical history, saving the physician time and leaving the present illness to the physician to develop during his conversation with the patient. Note that much of the actual chief complaint was captured by the questions in the system review part of the history. The patient's principle diagnoses: chronic bronchitis, hiatus hernia and hemorrhoids were strongly suspected by the medical history and were subsequently confirmed.

The end

978-0-595-42662-1
0-595-42662-X

Printed in the United States
109275LV00008B/50/A